# New Beginnings

Towards patient and public involvement in primary health care

# New Beginnings

Towards patient and public involvement in primary health care

Edited by Stephen Gillam and Fiona Brooks

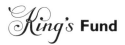

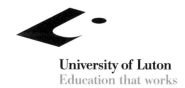

University of Luton
Education that works

Published by
King's Fund Publishing
11–13 Cavendish Square
London W1G 0AN

© King's Fund 2001

First published 2001

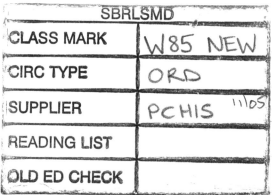
ISBN 1 85717 439 9

A CIP catalogue record for this book is available from the British Library

Available from:
King's Fund Bookshop
11–13 Cavendish Square
London
W1G 0AN

Tel:   020 7307 2591
Fax:   020 7307 2801

Printed and bound in Great Britain

*Cover photograph: John Birdsall Photography*

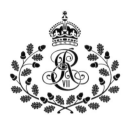

# Contents

## Part I Shaping public and patient involvement

## Part II User voices

# New Beginnings: towards patient and public involvement in primary health care

Foreword by Rabbi Julia Neuberger

Primary care is the hub of the NHS. It is in the human relationships between GPs, practice nurses, therapists and patients that the majority of health care is carried out in the UK. While medical miracles steal the headlines, what matters most for the majority of health service users is that they have access to health professionals who care, who empathise and who can be trusted.

Health care is, in essence, an activity in which human beings entrust their minds and bodies to people they believe will improve, maintain or protect them. It is an implicit contract between two people, both of whom need to be active participants to achieve effective outcomes. Yet the language of Western medicine has, for many decades, been one that assumes the health care relationship to be inherently unequal. The doctor, armed with medical science, is all-powerful, while the patient is essentially passive and, in the NHS, grateful for what he/she receives. The only involvement required in this model is to give consent to what is proposed, to comply with treatment regimes and to live more healthily in future.

That model, however, is losing its dominance. There is a growing body of evidence that patients who are involved in decisions about their treatment may get better outcomes from health care. There is more and more pressure on health systems to respond to users' views of their services, taking a more consumer-focused approach to their work. This pressure has increased considerably in the past two years, as trust in the medical profession takes one blow after another as the failings of a few are exposed in the mass media. In addition, as debates about the allocation of scarce resources for health care heat up, there is a need for citizens to make some of the trade-offs required of health services.

The case for greater public and user involvement is thus both practical and ethical. A twenty-first century health system simply cannot afford to ignore its users. At the primary care level, where good human relationships are essential to promote fair access to health care, the voices of patients, user groups, citizens and non-users must all be heard clearly by service providers.

User involvement can no longer be seen as a burdensome addition to primary care. It needs to become part and parcel of everyday practice. The Government's *NHS Plan* provides a sketchy outline of how the health service will become more responsive to patients and the public. The challenge for the people who have to enact *The NHS Plan* – essentially, the one million people who work for it – is to develop positive methods of public involvement that add to the value of the NHS. They need to ensure that individual patients, from all backgrounds, are empowered to make decisions about their health; that feedback from user groups really influences service provision; and that informed citizenship actively shapes primary care development. This is not an option – it is an imperative.

# Preface

User involvement in health forms a cornerstone of recent shifts in health policy, particularly those relating to the delivery of primary health care. The development of user involvement represents a challenging arena for health care professionals, demanding both new working practices as well as a radical shift in attitudes.

However, both theoretically and practically, user involvement represents something of a minefield. Approaching the field, the practitioner or student is faced with an array of terminology and methods across a spectrum of political philosophies. This is reflected in the diverse and somewhat unwieldy multi-disciplinary literature concerned with user participation in health services. This text is primarily intended to offer an accessible means of contextualising and analysing the complex issues surrounding user involvement. It does not set out to offer the reader a 'how to do user involvement' manual (Chambers, 2000) nor attempt to identify the 'best model'. Instead, the book offers a means of exploring the links between user involvement and improved quality of care.

The material presented in this book aims to illustrate the importance of user involvement for practitioners in their day-to-day interactions. In particular, we seek to provide a means of understanding the cultural and attitudinal change that is required of practitioners in order to achieve effective user involvement.

The text draws together recent applied research concerned with a wide range of user groups that has been undertaken by the King's Fund and the Institute for Health Services Research at the University of Luton. Through illustrative case studies, readers should be able to develop a critical understanding of the potential impact of user involvement on primary health care.

The first section of the book is concerned with the theoretical and policy contexts that are shaping user involvement in the UK. Chapter 1 is concerned with the *why* of user involvement, it examines the value of user involvement and indicates the range of methodologies available.

Chapter 2 considers user involvement within broader policy and historical contexts. Chapter 3 specifically explores user involvement in relation to Primary Care Groups/Trusts, while Chapter 4 considers the development of partnerships in the primary care consultation.

In Part II, *User Voices*, a wide range of researchers and practitioners take a case study approach and provide contributions that seek to illustrate the diversity of issues encompassed by attempting to involve users in the primary health care process.

Finally, the book concludes with an overview of the challenges remaining and provides an indication of how user involvement can be moved forward.

## A note on terminology – What's in a name?

Terminology in this area is problematic, in that available terms for people who encounter health systems are politically 'loaded' or describe different forms of relationship (Herxheimer and Goodare, 1999). The term 'patient' raises difficulties because it denotes passivity within a medicalised encounter and is not relevant for much of the preventive or health promotion work of primary health care. However, it is the most commonly understood and used term, and does allow for the vulnerable position of people when 'ill'. 'Consumer' and 'customer' have been largely discredited as they imply simplistic parallels between choices exercised in the health service sector. 'User' and 'client' can imply a formal relationship to the health services that may be inaccurate or misleading. 'Co-producer of health work' is valuable as a concept but cumbersome to use as a practical descriptor. The problematic nature of all the available terms leaves authors and practitioners in a quandary. In this text, we have generally opted for the most neutral of the available terms, that of 'users', while 'patients' is used by some authors in referring to clinical settings.

# References

Chambers R. *Involving patients and the public. How to do it better.* Abingdon: Radcliffe Medical Press, 2000.
Herxheimer A, Goodare H. Who are you and who are we? Looking through some key words. *Health Expectations* 1999; 2 (1): 3–6.

Fiona Brooks
Stephen Gillam
January 2001

# Notes on Contributors

## About the editors

**Fiona Brooks** is a medical sociologist and Deputy Director of the Institute for Health Services Research based at the University of Luton. She has a long-standing interest in the impact of policy developments on women's health care, including the policy implications of innovative service developments and user empowerment. She is currently leading a number of projects broadly concerned with governance in health systems, including an evaluation of a user-participation council.

**Stephen Gillam** is Director of the Primary Care Programme at the King's Fund and an honorary clinical senior lecturer in the Department of Primary Care and Population Sciences at the UCH Royal Free Medical School. He began his career in general practice before moving into public health medicine following a period overseas with the Save the Children Fund. He previously worked as a consultant in public health medicine for Bedfordshire Health Authority. He continues part-time clinical practice in Luton.

Both editors have published widely in the area of primary health care.

## Chapter authors

**Will Anderson** co-ordinates the London-wide evaluation of public involvement in Primary Care Groups at the King's Fund.

**Penny Banks** is a Fellow in the Health and Social Care Programme at the King's Fund.

**Angela Coulter** is the Chief Executive of Picker Institute Europe.

**Margaret Edwards** is the Project Manager for the Primary Care Groups and Older People Project at the King's Fund.

**Brian Fisher** is a general practitioner in south-east London and Clinical Director of South Lewisham PCG.

**Dominique Florin** is a Fellow in the Primary Care Programme at the King's Fund.

**David Gilbert** is a Senior Fellow at the Office of Public Management.

**Angela Greatley** is a Fellow in the Primary Care Programme (mental health) at the King's Fund.

**Helen Lomax** is a Research Fellow at the Institute for Health Services Research, University of Luton.

**Martin Mitchell** is a Research Fellow at the Institute for Health Services Research, University of Luton.

# Acknowledgements

The editors wish to thank their organisations, colleagues and families for their support. There is obviously a need for a collective thank-you to all the users and patients who contributed to the voices in the cases studies; we hope this text is true to their views and experiences.

# Part I

# Shaping public and patient involvement

Chapter 1

# Why user involvement in primary health care?

Fiona Brooks

**KEY POINTS**

■ Primary health care providers face a crossroads in their relationships with patients. They must create an effective dialogue with increasingly informed and critical users, or face conflict-ridden interactions and potentially greater levels of litigation.

■ The development of effective user involvement is not simply fashionable rhetoric but offers real potential for improved clinical outcomes and service development.

■ User involvement in health care decision-making is a dynamic process, one in which users' views are likely to become shaped by the process. Professionals need to value critical, reflective and informed service users in order to achieve user-centred service provision.

■ Moving from data collection to beneficial outcomes is the great challenge for user involvement in primary care. The essential issue is not a choice between different models but the creation of a change in professional attitudes and organisational culture.

## Section One: Why user involvement?

The greatest challenge for health services at the beginning of the twenty-first century is likely to be the achievement of effective patient and public involvement. Health service provision is in danger of being overwhelmed by the problems of ever increasing demand, resource prioritisation, increasing user litigation and resulting low professional morale. Incorporating the *user voice* and achieving a partnership with patients is being seen by policy-makers as one means of resolving these contested areas of health care delivery (Department of Health, 1999; Department of Health, 2000). Consequently, central to the array of policy and organisational changes being implemented in the NHS is the notion of making the service both more accountable to service users and more responsive to user definitions of need (Department of Health, 1999).

However, the notion that user involvement is a central component of an 'improved health service' is not new. User involvement in health services during the latter decades of the twentieth century has been an iconic vehicle for the presentation of differing welfare ideologies. In the health arena, user involvement has shifted from the idea of the patient as a consumer in an organisation driven by market forces (Department of Health and Social Security, 1983; Department of Health, 1989), to the view that participation is an essential ingredient of democratic and accountable services (Department of Health, 1999; Department of Health, 2000). Although representing diverse political philosophies, unifying all these interpretations is the goal of those trying to change the professional and organisational culture of the NHS.

Public and patient involvement is not only moving centre stage in all sectors of welfare provision; health service providers also face a crossroads in their relationship with patients. Cultural change, supported by new information and communication technologies, has altered user expectations of encounters with practitioners. In the consultation, patient passivity in the form of unquestioned deference or trust is being replaced with an expectation by users of agency in their encounters with professionals. In the broader public arena, notorious failures by practitioners in their duty to care have damaged public confidence (Dryer, 2000). Consequently, the NHS either creates an effective dialogue with increasingly informed and critical users, or faces conflict-ridden interactions and potentially greater levels of litigation.

Moreover, user involvement in primary care at both the level of individual care and service planning is relatively underdeveloped (Audit Commission, 1996). In moving towards more participatory approaches to the organisation and delivery of care, primary care professionals not only have to grapple with an attitudinal shift, but also lack tried and trusted models for the achievement of effective user involvement (Rummery and Glendinning, 2000).

## The value and benefits of patient expertise

The drive for user involvement should not be interpreted solely as a defensive reaction to user criticism, or fashionable packaging for policy and organisational change. Instead, the achievement of effective user involvement in primary care offers real potential for improved clinical outcomes.

In essence, user involvement in primary care can be viewed as occurring at two levels:

1. First, at the individual level – in the clinical encounter – service users and carers are involved in decisions concerning their treatment and care. This encompasses terms such as 'shared decision-making' and 'informed choice', and some forms of health promotion advice.

2. Second, with collective and representational forms of involvement. This may involve groups, communities or individual representatives in strategic decision-making, such as service commissioning and resource allocation. This may also involve users in monitoring service delivery or assessing quality of care as part of clinical governance.

Involvement in service planning has shown that service users are able to generate creative solutions and ideas that benefit the organisation as a whole (Seymour, 1997). At the level of individual care, shared decision-making has been found to result in better health outcomes, for example in the management of chronic conditions such as diabetes and asthma (Huygen *et al.* 1992; Stewart 1995; Lorig *et al.* 1999).

> *The concept of patients as partners is far from political correctness gone too far; it is essential for efficient doctor–patient consultations in which mutual understanding leads to rapid diagnosis and negotiated treatment options that are thus more likely to be adhered to.* (Slowie, 1999)

However, faced with increasing demands on the service, stretched practitioners can fall into a position of seeing patients as burdens, or 'heartsinks', with the result that a conflictual relationship is set in place. It then becomes difficult for the practitioner to develop creative improvements in the quality of care. In contrast, an effective partnership with patients offers real solutions to the increased demands placed on practitioners because of the additional resources patients bring to the consultation. At the individual level they bring their own situated and embodied knowledge, as well as their capacity for the maintenance and amelioration of their own and their families' health. Patients also bring expert knowledge of their local communities and of the health issues facing them, and of the communities' resources. Professionals rarely possess all the competencies and skills required to ensure a successful outcome; instead, these are distributed *between* service users and professionals (Young *et al.* 1998).

Many authors have argued for a re-conceptualisation by professionals and users of their relationship to one another in order to harness patients' expertise (Stacey, 1982; Graham, 1984; Øvretveit, 1997; Wensing and Grol, 1998). In order to understand the process whereby health is both restored and maintained, users of health services need to be viewed as 'health workers' or co-producers of health (Stacey, 1982; Hart, 1988). At the level of the consultation, the view of the user of health services as an unpaid health worker alters the boundaries of the consultation. The user is no longer a passive patient who receives health information from a professional, but a team member whose expert knowledge about his/her own health and well-being actively contributes to an effective resolution of the health problem. Such re-shaping of the consultation enables health care professionals to understand why there is often little concordance in the consultation and why service users frequently do not act on advice given by health care professionals. Moreover, to perceive the patient as a health worker immediately acknowledges that health care work occurs outside the consulting room. It also allows the professional to acknowledge the caring expertise held by members of the patient's social support network.

Exploration of the notion of users as having expertise that constitutes health work will be further explored in the later case study chapters. In particular, these chapters will highlight the value of including user expertise as part of the primary care process for both users and professionals, and the overall quality of service delivery.

# Section Two: User involvement – dilemmas and challenges

*There is a great deal of rhetoric about public participation but a marked unwillingness to really engage in the processes which bring it about.*
(Ashton and Seymour, 1988)

A central aim of this book is to explore the elements that underpin effective user involvement in primary health care. In so doing, the book seeks to challenge assumptions that patients or groups of patients lack the capacity to be involved in health care decision-making. While it is likely to remain a reality that some patients – through vulnerability, severity of illness or choice – will wish to leave the ultimate responsibility for decision-making to professionals, the extent of the desire for professional decision-making may be over-estimated. Studies have shown that users' desire and capacity for involvement in decision-making is higher than professionals often acknowledge. For example, mental health service users have been found to want involvement in the development of their services but have been blocked by professional protectionism (Glenister, 1994).

While the focus of this book is the attitudinal and organisational context required to achieve user involvement, this does not lessen the importance of user responsibility. With rights to decision-making come responsibilities for accepting the risk and outcomes of the decision (see Chapter 5 on women's health).

This book expands the definition of patient involvement as the provision of information *to* patients. This unidirectional model reinforces inequities between provider and service user without allowing patients to input their expert knowledge into the consultation. Instead, the chapters in this book suggest an alternative perspective: that is, to achieve effective user involvement, practitioners must develop a more sophisticated understanding of the obstacles to user involvement and, in particular, the inequities in that relationship (Beresford *et al.* 2000). However, it is worth taking a critical look at some of the central objections and barriers to user involvement in health care decision-making.

## Whose priorities count?

Effective user participation is centred on the user perspective, with the result that the control of decision-making shifts *towards* the user. This should not simply reform or humanise health care, but make substantive changes. It is the failure to achieve this alteration of the balance of power that provides the main reason why many initiatives attempting user involvement have failed. They have faltered because they attempted to incorporate user knowledge to support or develop organisational and professional priorities, rather than address the core concerns of users.

> *Service agency discourse, not surprisingly, is primarily concerned with policy and services; with service organisation, management, efficiency, effectiveness and economy ... Service users' discourse is concerned much more explicitly and specifically with peoples lives.* (Beresford et al. 2000)

The adoption of a user-centred approach necessitates an understanding of the competing nature of discourses, values and assumptions between health care organisations and users. Conversely, an absence of such an understanding frequently results in strategies that *consult* users on a pre-determined organisational or professional agenda, while demanding consistent commitment from users. In the latter context, user need is defined by professionals, and user involvement is often confined to a broad definition of public participation (Rhodes and Nocon, 1998).

> *Consultation and participation are the usual ways that power centres think of involving other people – but these are usually attempts to enrol others in support of the priorities and agendas of the power centres themselves, in support of their own initiatives.* (Wright, 1999)

This leads to problems of sustainability, as users begin to question the value and quality of user involvement initiatives; a criticism that may account for the short lifespan of many 'patient participation groups' in general practice (Brown, 1999).

However, health care and welfare organisations and policies are structured by competing organisational, political and professional discourses, that may generate organisational opposition (Stevenson and Parsloe, 1993). Primary care practitioners, in attempting to promote a user-centred approach, may also find themselves in conflict with the demands placed on them for efficiency and cost effectiveness.

## Equity

Taking user participation beyond the level of the individual consultation – to user or community involvement in planning and managing services – raises another contested area, that of equity in service provision. Some evidence from public and patient involvement projects has indicated that the involvement of users/patients in decision-making over the planning, organisation, delivery and resourcing of services may result in the reinforcement of inequities rather than their elimination. User groups have been found to be less concerned than professionals with issues of equity, and to deal with issues of resource allocation by limiting universal access to core and preventive services (Stronks *et al.* 1997). The needs of some groups may be marginalised by public or patient groups. For example, treatment for children has been given priority over services for the elderly and conditions considered to be related to health damaging behaviours, such as smoking (Bowling, 1996; Stronks *et al.* 1997).

However, participation in health care decision-making needs to be understood as an evolving process in which user views are being dynamically shaped by participation. Opportunities for discussion and reflection on the complex implications of priority setting in primary care have generated radical changes in people's views on issues of equity, resulting in less discrimination against individuals with health damaging behaviours (Dolan, 1999). In this respect, models such as citizens' juries – that create a dialogue by providing users with ways to input their own situated knowledge and also to gain access to organisational knowledge – are likely to be most effective (Davies, 2000).

In order to pursue equity in resource allocation, the means must be found to ensure an effective voice for less powerful, marginalised groups. Specifically, attempting to achieve equal broad-based participation may result in a failure to prioritise the high need possessed by some minority groups (Hopton, 1995). Socio-economic factors, institutional racism, time constraints, poverty and extreme vulnerability may all result in groups such as women, black and ethnic minority communities and the very ill being excluded from participation initiatives (Davey, 1999). At the level of the consultation, low involvement in decision-making and a lack of conversational symmetry in the interaction have been associated with medical practitioners labelling patients in terms of their own culturally-determined values (Fisher and Groce, 1985). Consequently, strategies to develop user involvement need to acknowledge that equity is unlikely to be achieved by attempting to give all groups or individuals an equal 'voice'. Instead, strategies need to be based on an understanding of the dynamics of differential power between users and providers, between groups of users, and between different groups of providers (O'Keefe and Hogg, 2000).

Consideration of differential power raises a number of questions. First, how can the 'articulation of voices for different groups' be achieved? One prominent example of such a strategy is Iris Young's (1990) notion of 'veto groups', whereby particular marginalised groups are provided with a separate forum as well as a right to a *veto* over the issues most directly of concern to them. Second, how can participation of minority voices be achieved without their physical presence at meetings/panels? This presents a complex problem of representation for PCGs and PCTs, as many of the models for involving users are dependent upon attendance from users in order to create a dialogue. An attendance requirement is very likely to disenfranchise users who lack the time or the physical, emotional or financial resources to participate.

## What ever happened to *grateful* patients?

User involvement has also been alleged to be counterproductive to good user–professional relationships. This critique takes several related forms, for example that:

1.  user involvement will raise expectations and create an increase in demand
2.  participation will result in a reduction in user satisfaction as users become more critical

3. users will make conservative decisions in relation to their own care and thereby prevent developments in medical treatment.

For example, an evaluation of increased information provision for patients referred for coronary angiography found that although patients became more knowledgeable they also became less satisfied with their treatment and, particularly, the decision-making process (Bernstein *et al.* 1998). This finding led the authors to question the value of such educational material, but interestingly not the quality of the physician counselling. Such sentiments may reflect professional paternalism. O'Connor *et al.* (1999), on the contrary, did not find that access to full information, including side effects, resulted in conservative treatment options being chosen.

Greater involvement in the delivery of their care is likely to lead to critical responses from service users, responses that should foster debate rather than being seen as problematic. The determination of the extent of involvement different users actually want is a problematic issue for health professionals and policy-makers alike (Coulter, 1999). If one of the goals of user involvement is the empowerment of individuals, families and communities, then a more critical, reflective service user is to be welcomed.

*Getting involved may not only lead to change, but also change us. We become different. We become 'unrepresentative' in ways some service providers do not want. We become confident, experienced, informed and effective.* (Beresford and Campbell, 1994)

Will user involvement raise expectations and create an increase in demand? User empowerment may actually function to contain costs through improvements in efficiency by users generating innovative solutions to organisational and care problems (Wennberg, 1984). User participation is not, of course, an alternative to adequate resourcing of health services (Barnes and Walker, 1996). If user involvement were sought solely to reduce demand, then users would question the ethical base of their involvement, and the conflictual nature of user–provider relationships would be likely to intensify. Moreover, it is somewhat patronising to assume that the majority of users are unaware of the limited nature of resources for service provision (Barnes and Walker, 1996).

## Section Three: The 'how' of user involvement

### Information, participation and empowerment

User involvement constitutes a wide range of practices and user–provider relationships, the meanings and definitions of which are also contested and evolving (Warren, 1999). The models of user involvement are often conceptualised as a form of continuum, with information provision and health education at the lower end of the scale, and participation and empowerment at the higher end (Poulton, 1999). Participation is concerned with democratic decision-making in that the user – either at the individual or community level – negotiates with providers and influences the nature of service provision (Barnes and Wistow, 1992). Empowerment is seen as a development of participation in that the user gains power over the decision-making process and is able to effectively advance his/her own agenda (Davey, 1999). Information-giving alone can be criticised for being 'linear' (solely from the practitioner to the user) and maintaining user passivity, whereas improving access to information is a necessary element of effective participation. Examples of improved access to information include the usable information produced for citizens' juries or, at the individual level, enabling users to find pathways through the array of clinical information to make an appropriate treatment choice for their needs.

### Methodologies and methods of involving users

In practice, a vast array of approaches and tools has at some time been used to enable user involvement. Some represent actual research data-collection tools such as focus groups and in-depth interviews, while others such as citizens' juries, patient-participation groups or patient panels are methodologies designed solely to address user participation. Table 1.1 provides an overview of the main methodologies for eliciting users' and communities' collective views. Later chapters in the book will explore the practical realities of implementing approaches to user participation, while Florin and Coulter explore participation in the consultation. Debates over the most appropriate methodology can obscure essential challenges that all models face in creating outcomes that are of benefit to users.

**Table 1.1** Overview of main methods for obtaining user and communities views

| Method | Strengths | Weaknesses |
|---|---|---|
| **Structured questionnaires,** e.g. patient satisfaction surveys. | Relatively low cost. Potential for large sample population. Not too demanding of users' time. | Question design and analysis requires considerable methodological expertise. Relatively low level of user knowledge and expertise tapped. Users rarely involved in setting the focus and design of the questions. |
| **Qualitative techniques,** e.g. semi-structured in-depth interviews, focus groups. | Can allow for users' own agenda and priorities to emerge, rather than responding only to questions set by professionals. Useful methods for exploring the experiences of particular groups of users such as minority groups. Highly effective for exploring sensitive and complex issues. Focus groups useful for eliciting how groups of users rank priorities. | Focus groups are a fashionable methodology and not always used appropriately. Question construction and the conduct of the techniques is a skilled craft, particularly if issues of bias are to be handled effectively. Collection and analysis of the data is costly and time consuming. Also requires more time from users than a survey. |

| Method | Strengths | Weaknesses |
|---|---|---|
| **Consultation exercises,** e.g. public meetings, public opinion exercises. | May employ a variety of methods to gain users' views. Public support may improve the speed of change. | Often fails to reach the majority of the population. Often used to justify or 'explain' professional and organisational decisions. No clear link from users' voice to decision-making process. |
| **User representation,** e.g. on PCGs, citizens' juries, user panels, patient councils, patient-participation groups. | Aims to achieve a direct link between user expertise and the planning and delivery of services. Likely to develop the expertise and knowledge base of those involved. | Can create an empowered, informed elite. Issues of the breadth and appropriateness of representation. Views of participants can be disregarded by commissioning body. |
| **Community development** | Enables a means of addressing the broad social and economic causes of health inequalities. Seeks to empower and create community responses to health needs. Increases the 'social capital' within a community. | In practice, users/communities have not always been involved in determining priorities and resource allocation. Long-term outcomes are difficult to measure, which may make funding difficult to secure. |

All too often users provide time, ideas and expertise, only to see their contribution fail to materialise into actual change (Barnes and Walker, 1996). Although representing a start in a process, the collection of data using postal surveys and focus groups does not constitute actual involvement in decision-making. Similarly, many consultations, even where they ostensibly invite discussion, are in reality merely exercises in seeking user validation for pre-determined decisions (Chambers, 2000).

For user expertise and situated knowledge to be incorporated into practice, involvement in the construction and development of health knowledge will be important. This means that users will need to be directly involved in the setting of research agendas and questions. The involvement of users in the research process is still often limited, at best, to feedback of findings or representation on steering committees.

Ultimately, it is the intended purpose of user involvement that will largely determine the model adopted (Hickey and Kipping, 1998). To move beyond professional and organisational agendas requires not only the motivation to improve the quality of services, but also a strategy to enhance the capacity of users to participate in decisions concerning the organisation of services (Barnes and Wistow, 1992).

## References

Ashton J, Seymour H. *The New Public Health*. Buckingham: Open University, 1988.

Audit Commission. *What the doctor ordered: A study of GP fundholders in England and Wales*. London: HMSO, 1996.

Barnes M, Walker A. Consumerism versus empowerment: A principles approach to the involvement of older service users. *Policy and Politics* 1996; 24 (4): 375–93.

Barnes M, Wistow G. Understanding user involvement. In: Barnes M, Wistow G, editors. *Researching user involvement*. Leeds: Nuffield Institute for Health, University of Leeds, 1992.

Beresford P, Campbell J. Disabled people, service users, user involvement and representation. *Disability and Society* 1994; 9 (3): 315–25.

Beresford P, Croft S, Evans C, Harding T. Quality in personal social services: The developing role of user involvement in the UK. In: Davies C, Finlay L, Bullman A, editors. *Changing practice in health and social care*. London: Sage, 2000.

Bernstein S, Skarupski K, Grayson C, Starling M, Bates E, Eagle K. A randomized controlled trail of information-giving to patients referred for coronary angiography: effects on outcomes of care. *Health Expectations* 1998; (1): 50–61.

Bowling A. Health Care Rationing: the public's debate. *BMJ* 1996; 312: 670–74.

Brown I. Patient participation groups in general practice in the National Health Service. *Health Expectations* 1999; 2 (3): 169–78.

Chambers R. *Involving patients and the public. How to do it better.* Abingdon: Radcliffe Medical Press, 2000.

Coulter A. Paternalism or Partnership? Editorial. *BMJ* 1999; 319: 719–20.

Davey B. Solving economic, social and environmental problems together: an empowerment strategy for losers. In: Barnes M, Warren L, editors. *Paths to empowerment.* Bristol: The Policy Press, 1999.

Davies C. Frameworks for regulation and accountability: threat or opportunity? In: Brechin A, Brown H, Eby M, editors. *Critical practice in Health and Social Care.* London: Sage, 2000: 296–317.

Department of Health. *NHS & Community Care Act.* London: HMSO, 1989.

Department of Health. *Patient and public involvement in the new NHS.* London: HMSO, 1999.

Department of Health. *The NHS Plan. A plan for investment. A plan for reform.* London: HMSO, 2000.

Department of Health and Social Security. *Inquiry into NHS Management. (The Griffiths Report).* London: HMSO, 1983.

Dolan P. Effect of discussion and deliberation on the public's views of priority setting in health care: focus group study. *BMJ* 1999; 318: 916–19.

Dryer C. Tighter controls on GPs to follow doctor's murder convictions. *BMJ* 2000; 320: 331.

Fisher S, Groce S. Doctor–patient negotiation of cultural assumptions. *Sociology of Health and Illness* 1985; 7 (3): 342–74.

Glenister D. Patient participation in psychiatric services: a literature review and proposal for a research strategy. *Journal of Advanced Nursing* 1994; 19: 802–11.

Graham H. *Women, Health and the Family.* London: Harvester Press, 1984.

Hart J T. *A New Kind of Doctor.* London: Merlin Press, 1988.

Hickey G, Kipping C. Exploring the concept of user involvement in mental health through a participation continuum. *Journal of Clinical Nursing* 1998; 7: 83–88.

Hopton J. Patients' perceptions of need for primary health care services: useful for priority setting? *BMJ* 1995; 310: 1237–40.

Huygen F, Mokkink H, Smits A *et al.* Relationship between the working styles of general practitioners decision-making styles. *Ann. Intern. Med.* 1996; 124: 497–504.

Lorig K *et al.* Evidence suggesting that a chronic disease self-management programme can improve health status while reducing hospitalization: a randomized trial. *Med. Care* 1999; 37 (1): 5–14.

O'Connor A, Rostom A, Fiset V, Tetroe J, Entwistle V, Llewellyn-Thomas H, Holmes-Rovner M, Barry M, Jones J. Decision aids for patients facing health treatment or screening decisions: systematic review. *BMJ* 1999; 319: 731–34.

O'Keefe E, Hogg C. Public participation and maginalized groups: the community development model. *Health Expectations* 2000; 2 (4): 245–54.

Øvretveit J. How patient power and client participation affects relations between professions. In: Øvretveit J, Mathias P, Thompson T, editors. *Interprofessional working for health and social care.* London: Macmillan, 1997.

Poulton B. (1999) User involvement in identifying health needs and shaping and evaluation services: is it being realised? *Journal of Advanced Nursing* 1999; 30 (6): 1289–96.

Rhodes P, Nocon A. User involvement and the NHS reforms. *Health Expectations* 1998; 1 (2): 73–78.

Rummery K, Glendinning C. *Primary Care and Social Services: Developing new partnerships for older people.* Abingdon: National Primary Care Research and Development Series, Radcliffe Medical Press, 2000.

Seymour J. Patient Counselling. *Health Management* 1997; June: 14–17.

Slowie D F. Doctors should help patients to communicate better with them. *BMJ* 1999; 319: 784.

Stacey M. *Who are the health workers? Patients and other unpaid workers in health care.* Mexico: Paper presented at the ISA Conference, 1982.

Stevenson O, Parsloe P. *Community care and empowerment.* York: Joseph Rowntree Foundation, 1993.

Stewart M. Effective patient–physician communication and health outcomes: A review. *Journal of the Canadian Medical Association* 1995; 152 (9): 1423–33.

Stronks K, Strijbis A-M, Wendte J F, Gunning-Schepers L. Who should decide? Qualitative analysis of panel data from public, patients, healthcare professionals, and insurers on priorities in health care. *BMJ* 1997; 315: 92–96.

Warren L. Conclusion: empowerment: the path to partnership? In: Barnes M, Warren L, editors. *Paths to empowerment.* Bristol: The Policy Press, 1999.

Wennberg J. Dealing with medical practice variations: a proposal for action. *Health Affairs* 1984; (4) 3: 6–32.

Wensing M, Grol R. What can patients do to improve health care? *Health Expectations* 1998; 1: 37–49.

Wright A. Exploring the development of user forums in an NHS trust. In: Barnes M, Warren L, editors. *Paths to empowerment.* Bristol: The Policy Press, 1999.

Young A, Ackerman J, Kyle J. *Looking on: Deaf People and the Organisation of Services*. Bristol: The Policy Press, 1998.

Young I. Polity and group difference. In: Young I, editor. *Throwing like a girl and other essays in feminist philosophy*. Bloomington: Indiana University Press, 1990.

Chapter 2

# Primary care: evolving policy

Stephen Gillam

### KEY POINTS

■ A succession of reforms has done little to increase public and patient involvement in the running of the health service.

■ The information revolution is making new demands of health professionals and changing traditional power relations with patients.

■ Policies designed to increase access to primary care may compromise the continuity and co-ordination of care that users also value.

■ Personal lists and traditional referral arrangements underpin the efficiency of the NHS but are increasingly seen as constraining for users.

## Introduction

Increasing patient or user involvement has been a common preoccupation of successive governments over the last twenty years. The language and terminology may have changed but the challenges have not. A brief historical detour into the roots of general practice helps explain some of its enduring strengths and its weaknesses as currently perceived, before considering what we know about what matters to users and patients now. Consideration is then given to the reforms initiated by the Labour government since 1997. The impact of new information technologies and the proliferation of access routes to primary care are also explored. The chapter finishes with reference to the implications of the recent *NHS Plan*.

## History – the foundations of general practice

The profession of general practice derived over the course of the nineteenth century from the trade of apothecaries. In the growing industrial cities where GPs relied on patients' fees, nobody was seen in the out-patient clinics of charitable hospitals unless referred by a GP.

This was the origin of the first of three fundamental principles of general practice in the UK, that of referral, whereby GPs became the 'gate-keepers' to secondary care (Hannay *et al.* 2000).

The second principle concerns non-specialisation, since most scientific advances and medical care took place in hospitals. Even now, intriguingly, evidence suggests that for many people 'primary care' means hospital care (Pedersen *et al.* 1998). However, the evolution of the 'expert generalist', able to co-ordinate the management of patients from the centre of a web of health professionals, is seen as a source of the NHS' efficiency.

By the beginning of the twentieth century, GPs were increasingly being paid an insurance fee by patients as members of 'sick clubs'. These were the forerunner of the National Insurance Act 1911, which covered wage earners and was extended to the whole population with the creation of the NHS in 1948. This provides the basis of the third principle: that of a capitation fee for everyone on a registered list of patients.

While the postgraduate training and professional development of British general practitioners became increasingly sophisticated, many countries saw the status of family practice decline. International comparisons of the extent to which health systems are primary care orientated suggests that those countries with more generalist family doctors acting as gate-keepers with registered lists are more likely to have better health outcomes as well as lower costs and greater satisfaction (Starfield, 1994). But if the British NHS remains one of the most efficient health systems in the world, these three key principles are increasingly seen as constraining.

Referral arrangements are now seen as monopolistic and restrictive. Many of this government's health policies have been designed to increase access to care through routes other than general practice (see below). The generalist is under threat. How can any single health professional stay abreast of advances in all branches of medical science? The personal list, coupled with doctors' sense of 'womb-to-tomb' round-the-clock responsibility in the traditions of Dr Finlay, has provided the bedrock of family practice for generations. The same dated model can be seen as one source of professional paternalism. But what do we really know about what matters to users and patients today?

## Public views

The public consistently attach highest priority to three particular facets of general practice (Greenhalgh *et al.* 1999). They want a personal relationship with someone who communicates well and who understands them. This underscores the importance of continuity of care. Second, they need to know that their doctor is technically sound in clinical terms. Third, they want to be able to rely on their general practitioner as a source of information, as someone with whom they can share decision-making.

The public may not use the term 'primary care' but they do relate to their general practice, and there is plenty of evidence to suggest that levels of satisfaction with general practice remain high. The methodological limitations of 'patient satisfaction' as a concept are widely recognised (Locker *et al.* 1987). Nevertheless, patient satisfaction surveys are reassuringly consistent. They suggest that the majority of patients are happy with the service they receive, but that difficulty gaining access is a growing concern, particularly for people from minority ethnic groups (NHS Executive, 1999). They also reveal consistent generational differences, with people aged over 65 years broadly more satisfied than younger people (Malbon *et al.* 1999). This may in part be a 'cohort effect' with greater support for the NHS evinced among those old enough to remember what preceded it. It is more likely to relate to changing needs. With age and the onset of chronic conditions, instant access may become less important than personal care.

The NHS remains popular as an institution for what it symbolises (Mulligan, 1997/8) – a central part of the social fabric to which public and politicians alike remain committed. Yet the corporate altruism of the post-war period that gave rise to the Welfare State can no longer be taken for granted. Nor can a utilitarian commitment to universal coverage. Support for a state-controlled system and the notion of a 'public service' ethos has steadily eroded under a growing combination of pressures. These include rising consumerism, technological advance and demographic change – the forces that have ensured that demand for health services steadily outstrips supply. These pressures have faced the NHS since its inception fifty years ago; others have intensified more recently.

Doctors and nurses may retain public respect, but in terms of social status, pay and professional autonomy they have been steadily losing ground. In an information-rich society, health professionals can no longer lay claim to being the only repository of knowledge. They are still struggling to come to terms with this shift in power relations. Day by day, loss of trust is reflected in rising levels of complaints and increasingly frequent litigation. The public expectations continue to outstrip the health system's capacity to deliver change and, in particular, to increase access. However, trust is multifaceted. The public seem able to distinguish these aspects of trust from those that derive from personal relationships with individuals moulded over time.

## Policy preoccupations

Over the last two decades consistent themes have preoccupied policy-makers: the need to contain rising health care costs, the desire to address variations in the quality of clinical care and the concern to make the service more responsive to consumers' needs, in particular regarding increased access.

The cost efficiency of the NHS, as we have seen, has long been attributed in large measure to general practice. The tripartite division between hospital, community and family practitioner services, with open access to family practitioner services but controlled access to specialist services, has endured since 1948. However, the very existence of this tripartite structure, combined with the independent contractor status of GPs, has resulted in a service that suffers from problems of poor communication and co-ordination, an inability to plan comprehensive services designed to address health needs, and wide variations in provision. Successive governments have become increasingly aware of the need to constrain costs and introduce incentives to improve quality. The reforms introduced by the Conservative government in 1990 concentrated on controlling cost and quality through the introduction of an internal market (Secretary of State for Health, 1989). One implicit justification for fundholding was that general practitioners were the most appropriate health professionals to judge the quality and balance of local service provision: best placed, if not best equipped, to act as advocates for their patients.

Although the proponents of GP fundholding claimed great benefits from the scheme, the evidence to support these claims is equivocal (Le Grand *et al.* 1998). The Audit Commission concluded that, apart from a small number of notable exceptions, most fundholding practices had produced only modest improvements and that these were probably insufficient to justify their higher cost (Audit Commission, 1996). Fundholding was judged a failure for several reasons. It was bureaucratic, involving high transaction costs. It was perceived as unfair: (successful) fundholders generated inequities in access to care (two-tierism). Most importantly, the internal market failed to deliver anticipated efficiency gains. Certainly, there was limited evidence that fundholding increased user involvement or choice (Le Grand *et al.* 1998). For example, patients were no more likely to exercise discretion in their choice of general practitioner. Yet it did entrench political support for widening the involvement of general practitioners in resource allocation.

## The New NHS

The publication of the Labour government's White Paper *The New NHS: modern, dependable* (Department of Health, 1997) formally announced the demise of GP fundholding and the internal market. However, the agenda set out in the White Paper was potentially far more radical than the abolition of market mechanisms. It underlined the role of the NHS in improving health, set out a renewed commitment to equity in access and provision, and tackled the need to ensure quality through clinical governance and accountability to local communities. Of fundamental importance was the move to loosen the restrictions of the old tripartite structure by moving towards unified budgets and imposing a duty of partnership with local authorities. The major structural change introduced to deliver these policy goals was the formation of Primary Care Groups (PCGs), with the expectation that these would, in due course, mature into freestanding Primary Care Trusts (PCTs). PCGs are expected to undertake three principal functions on behalf of their local populations:

- to improve the health of the population and address health inequalities
- to develop primary and community health services
- to commission a range of community and hospital services.

PCG/Ts bring together local providers of primary and community services under a board representing local GPs, nurses, the local community, social services and the health authority. PCG/Ts are required to engage the populations they serve in their decision-making procedures as they take responsibility for priority setting. This is a political process, for there remains no ethically coherent, scientific system for resolving debates about rationing.

## Clinical governance

Many public sector bodies have sought over the last ten years to import the organisation-wide quality-improvement strategies perceived as successful in manufacturing and service industries. The invention of clinical governance heralded the latest of many attempts in the NHS to exercise greater managerial control over clinical activities. It has been defined as a system through which NHS organisations are accountable for continuously improving the quality of their services and safeguarding high standards of care by creating an environment in which clinical excellence will flourish (NHS Executive, 1998).

Clinical governance is a system that draws together elements of quality assurance that are often ill co-ordinated. The corporate nature of this new responsibility requires, in the over-used phrase, major 'cultural change'. For PCGs, this implies sharing intelligence about quality across professional and practice boundaries, and health professionals seeing themselves as collectively accountable for the clinical and cost effectiveness of their colleagues' work.

Clinical governance is the glue that binds together a national framework (see Figure 2.1) in which two new bodies have central roles. The National Institute of Clinical Excellence is setting standards and

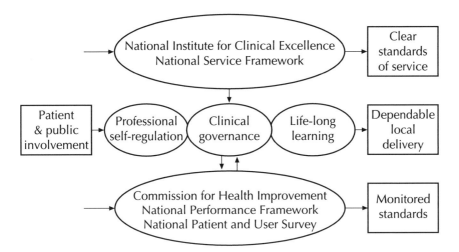

**Figure 2.1** A first class service

guiding the development of National Service Frameworks. The Commission for Health Improvement is responsible for monitoring implementation and for undertaking regular visits to assess the performance of the new primary care organisations. Clinical governance links critically to the processes of continuous professional development and is supposed to involve users. It also implies a new understanding about the nature of professional accountability. However, much of the focus of clinical governance in the early stages of its implementation has been on the management of poor performance. Quality assurance needs to be balanced by more supportive forms of professional development if professional morale is not to be needlessly damaged. Moreover, there is as yet little evidence of public involvement in the processes of clinical governance (Wilkin *et al.* 2000).

**Information and the balance of power**
Traditionally, medicine has been based on knowledge acquired during training and topped up from time to time from sources such as scientific journals, conferences and medical libraries. These dated quickly, but clinicians nevertheless had more knowledge than their patients who were denied access to such sources. However, as Muir Gray points out, 'The World Wide Web, the dominant medium of the postmodern world, has blown away the doors and walls of the locked library as efficiently as

Semtex' (Muir Gray, 1999). Admittedly, the quality of knowledge is variable, but that is changing. Increasingly, patients will be more knowledgeable than their doctors. For medicine to make the best of the information revolution, it must address three key issues: the use of informed choice as an outcome; the use of computers to repersonalise clinical practice; and the empowerment of patients.

As people gain access to information about risk, a higher proportion may choose not to accept the offer of screening or treatment. In the past, mortality reduction and population coverage were the criteria used to evaluate screening programmes. In future, measures of informed choice will also be needed.

The computer screen certainly threatens the interpersonal nature of the consultation. However, it is no longer necessary for clinicians to have to remember so many drug details or management indications. It is no wonder that patients complain about depersonalised care when clinicians are so preoccupied with technical aspects of their job. A range of new tools is available to deliver knowledge during a consultation. These tools can help change clinicians from seeking to be repositories of knowledge to being managers of knowledge.

Some clinicians are nervous of giving patients better information and not all patients want it (Street, 1997). However, most people want to be in charge of decisions about their health. There is evidence that the empowerment of patients, for example by giving them more knowledge or a consultation style that facilitates involvement, improves not only patient satisfaction but also clinical outcomes (Street, 1997). Patient involvement in the clinical encounter and the nature of shared decision-making are discussed by Dominique Florin and Angela Coulter in Chapter 4.

Medicine is not an exact science. Paradoxically, too heavy an emphasis on evidence-based medicine, guidelines and protocols may rob clinical practice of some of the responsiveness and flexibility that patients most value. The growing popularity of complementary therapies is testimony to anti-rationalism and the importance attached to holistic models of care.

# Access

National consumer satisfaction surveys have consistently found difficulties booking appointments, and waiting times for routine or emergency care, to be of public concern. A raft of new policy initiatives has been designed to improve access to primary care. The purpose of NHS Direct, the national nurse-led telephone helpline, is to provide 'easier and faster advice and information for people about health, illness and the NHS so that they are better able to care for themselves and their families'. But NHS Direct is more than a response to the consumerist demands of the '24-hour society'. More specific objectives include the encouragement of self-care at home and reducing unnecessary use of other NHS services – i.e. the management of demand (Rosen *et al.* 1999).

Both NHS Direct and the new walk-in centres involve forms of nurse triage. Some of the new practices, established using Personal Medical Services flexibilities, are effectively 'nurse-led' (Lewis *et al.* 1999). These innovations are changing the way primary care is perceived. In addition, a growing proportion of new entrants to general practice are women seeking to reconcile career aspirations with family responsibilities. Greater feminisation of the primary care workforce will alter the status and image of family doctoring. Health professionals fear that a plurality of access points could result in fragmented care. But the trade-off implied between personal continuity and modern care can be exaggerated. It is more often between small (more familiar) teams and large (more cost-efficient) ones. PCGs may offer the opportunity to separate administrative and clinical functions that work best on different scales (Guthrie *et al.* 2000).

# New Labour, new Plan

That general practitioners will prove capable of cost-effective stewardship of the NHS remains an article of faith. Labour's was allegedly a ten-year project, but the development of effective Primary Care Trusts was always going to take more time than the electoral cycle allowed. Similarly, the implementation of clinical governance was never going to keep health scandals from the national news. Prime ministerial frustration at the slow pace of modernisation was understandable. *The NHS Plan*, which defines the agenda for another Labour government, was one result (NHS Executive, 2000).

It was preceded by an extraordinary 'census' to try and define how the public would spend moneys pledged for the NHS. The polling exercise was criticised as undermining just those integrated and inclusive approaches to public involvement the Department of Health has sought to promote. In contrast to 'policymaking by 12 million leaflets' (Anderson and Florin, 2000), international examples have shown that meaningful consultation is complex and expensive (McKee *et al.* 1996). Regardless of whether the Plan's authors could claim greater democratic legitimacy, what does it presage for users of primary care?

Patients are to receive more information, for example about their practice (size, accessibility, performance against National Service Framework standards – the feared 'league tables'). There is to be a new patient advocacy service, new independent local advisory forums and reconfiguration panels. These developments are designed to bring patients and citizens into decision-making at every level of the service. The following chapter considers their likely impact in more detail. They form just one part of the drive to increase professional accountability. Health professionals were already bracing themselves for annual appraisals and mandatory audit in support of revalidation (NHS Executive, 1999). They have reason to fear the tightening noose of professional accountability. The loss of struggling colleagues and the time out needed to participate in continuing professional development will increase workloads. It remains to be seen whether these changes reassure the public.

The expansion in hospital beds and consultant numbers with consequent reductions in waiting times, if realised, will ease the burden of containment in primary care. The 3.4 per cent expansion in GP numbers is less impressive. Even allowing for investment in other community-based services, GPs will not easily be able to improve access to their services or extend consultation lengths. The Plan proposes further integration of NHS Direct and GP out-of-hours services. The vision is of a single phone call to NHS Direct as the one-stop gateway to all out-of-hours health care.

## Conclusion

*For the first time patients will have a real say in the NHS. They will have new powers and more influence over the way the NHS works.* (NHS Executive, 2000)

*The NHS Plan* reaffirms this government's commitment to strengthen user participation in the running of the NHS even if much of the document feels like 'more of the same'. In other respects this government's first four years have proved unexpectedly radical. The cost efficiency of the NHS has long been attributed in large measure to the strengths of British general practice, key features of which are the provision of continuous care and a comprehensive financing system. Both are under threat. How Primary Care Groups are taking up the challenge to involve users is considered by Will Anderson in the following chapter.

New Labour has staked its reputation on reform of the NHS but there are obvious dangers in continually fuelling public expectations. From the perspective of primary care professionals, nothing in the latest proposals tries to limit demand. Paradoxically, from the users' perspective, this government could yet break the NHS under the weight of its good intentions.

## References

Anderson W, Florin D. Consulting the public about the NHS. *BMJ* 2000; 320: 1553–54.

Audit Commission. *What the Doctor Ordered: a Study of GP Fundholding in England and Wales*. London: HMSO, 1996.

De Maeseneer J, Hjortdahl P, Starfield B. Fix what's wrong, not what's right, with general practice in Britain. *BMJ* 2000; 320: 1616–67.

Department of Health. *The New NHS: modern, dependable*. London: The Stationery Office, 1997.

Greenhalgh P, Eversley J. *Quality in General Practice*. London: King's Fund, 1999.

Guthrie B, Wyke S. Does continuity in general practice really matter? *BMJ* 2000; 321: 734–35.

Hannay D, Mathers N. General Practice, Management Culture and Market Ideology – Bedfellows or Culture Clash? *Brit. J. Gen. Pract.* 2000; 455: 518–19.

Le Grand J, Mays N, Mulligan J, editors. *Learning from the NHS Internal Market. A review of the evidence.* London: King's Fund, 1998.

Lewis R, Gillam S, editors. *Transforming Primary Care. Personal medical services in the new NHS.* London: King's Fund, 1999.

Locker D, Dunt D. Theoretical and methodological issues in sociological studies in consumer satisfaction with medical care. *Soc. Sci. Med.* 1987; 12: 283–92.

Malbon G, Jenkins C, Gillam S. *What do Londoners think of their general practice?* London: King's Fund, 1999.

McKee M, Figueras J. Setting priorities: can Britain learn from Sweden? *BMJ* 1996; 312: 691–94.

Muir Gray J A. Postmodern medicine. *Lancet* 1999; 354: 1550–53.

Mulligan J. Attitudes towards the NHS and its alternatives, 1983–96. In: *Health Care UK 1997/8.* London: King's Fund: 198–209.

NHS Executive. *A First Class Service: quality in the new NHS.* London: Department of Health, 1998.

NHS Executive. *National surveys of NHS patients. General practice 1998.* London: Department of Health, 1999.

NHS Executive. *Supporting Doctors, Protecting Patients.* London: Department of Health, The Stationery Office, 1999.

NHS Executive. *The NHS Plan. A plan for investment. A plan for reform.* Cm 4818-I. London: The Stationery Office, 2000.

Pedersen L L, Wilkin D. Primary health care: definitions, users and uses. *Health Care Anal.* 1998, 6 December (4): 341–51.

Rosen R, Florin D. Evaluating NHS Direct. *BMJ* 1999; 319: 5–6.

Secretary of State for Health. *Working For Patients.* London: HMSO, Cm 555.78, 1989.

Starfield B. Is primary care essential? *Lancet* 1994; 344: 1129–33.

Street R L, Voigt B. Patient participation in deciding breast cancer treatment and subsequent quality of life. *Med. Decis. Making* 1997; 17: 298–306.

Wilkin D, Gillam S, Leese B, editors. *The National Tracker Survey of Primary Care Groups and Trusts. Progress and Challenges 1999/2000.* London: National Primary Care Research and Development Centre/King's Fund, 2000.

Chapter 3

# Primary care groups: corporate opportunities for public involvement

Will Anderson

## KEY POINTS

■ Primary Care Groups (PCGs) have provided a new corporate focus for public involvement in primary care, particularly in the planning, development and monitoring of services.

■ Lay members have played a crucial role, but the paucity and fragmentation of national guidance on public involvement has left local development dependent on local commitments and skills.

■ Although public involvement is a commitment of many of the officers and members of PCGs, the demands of the development agenda and lack of resources have inhibited progress.

■ Public involvement initiatives are typically pursued with multiple objectives and sustained by diverse values and ideologies. Maximising the value of this diversity is the greatest challenge for PCGs.

■ Primary Care Trusts (PCTs) should provide opportunities to give greater institutional weight to public involvement in primary care.

## Introduction

Primary Care Groups (PCGs) were established in April 1999 as a cornerstone of the new government's commitment to creating a primary care-led NHS (Secretary of State, 1997). The last chapter explored the policy background that gave political credibility to the idea of primary care professionals leading not only the development of primary care but also the commissioning of secondary and community health services, and the 'health improvement' of the local population. This chapter explores how PCGs have addressed lay, user and public involvement, drawing on data from a recent King's Fund survey of the lay members and chief executives of PCGs in London (Anderson, 2000).

## A new player in the local health economy

PCGs have presented real opportunities for the development of user and public involvement in primary care. Not only are they new, they also have an explicit developmental mission – established to take forward a range of issues that have never before had a fully-fledged corporate focus in primary care. Public involvement is not the top priority of PCG boards, but nor has the issue been completely marginalised. In London, 63 per cent of PCG chief executives reported that there was a designated subgroup or working group with a brief for public involvement, and a further 21 per cent said there were plans to establish one. Furthermore, 91 per cent of PCGs had strategies for public involvement or plans to produce one. It is still early days, but these simple organisational indicators suggest that corporate commitment to public involvement is emerging within many PCGs.

If PCGs provide new opportunities for public involvement, these are nonetheless circumscribed by their place in local health economies and the extent of their influence and powers. User and public involvement in the NHS includes the individual treatment and care decisions of patients and carers, the user contribution to planning and monitoring services, and the citizen contribution to policy-making (Barnes and McIver, 1999). PCGs ought to be interested in all three of these levels of involvement, but in practice it is the second that has dominated their interests, reflecting their position between the front-line activity of Primary Health Care Teams (PHCTs) and the strategic and political decision-making of central government and health authorities.

Traditional professional–patient relationships have been shifting towards greater patient-centred practice for some time, driven by factors such as the patient role in treatment management and the value of patient perspectives in assessing quality (Rogers and Popay, 1997). Clinical governance now provides the framework by which PCGs can systematically address quality in the delivery of primary care. However, PCGs are still struggling with the profound organisational development challenges of working corporately with their constituent practices on such issues (Huntingdon, 2000). Public involvement in clinical governance is a novelty with few existing roots in Primary Health Care Teams (Allen, 2000).

Patient involvement in general practice has traditionally focused on collective action to support the work of practice, epitomised in patient-participation groups. The extent of this kind of involvement is easy to underestimate as it does not conform to the 'public meeting' image of involvement (Winkler, 1996). Although practices ought to provide great opportunities for community development (Fisher *et al.* 1999), this requires a long view and sustained support. PCGs that want to see more immediate results from involvement have turned to those things over which they have more direct control. Consequently, most public involvement initiatives have focused on the corporate concerns of the PCG itself.

> *I've got a session with a small practices group soon around community participation and that feels good, because it feels like that's where we really need to reach. I'm really thinking, 'Well, what might it mean for GPs, what might we do that's meaningful for GPs and patients?' I have to say I think it's about clinical governance – stuff to do with the relationship that you have with the person, you know, whether you listen. In a way, if I could get the GPs to be thinking about asking people what they think, that would be a pretty good start, because it doesn't happen now.*
>
> lay member

At the other end of the spectrum, PCGs want to take their responsibilities to their local populations seriously – to engage with citizens as well as users. They are better placed to do this than PHCTs, for whom the tension between the individual focus of the practice list population and the collective focus of the community as a whole may be an obstacle (Brown, 1994). However, given that strategic policy-making is likely to be dominated by the directives of health authorities and the NHS Executive, any involvement in local decision-making has to take seriously the limitations imposed from above. This tension between the implementation of national policy and meaningful local involvement in policy-making is a long-standing problem (Winkler, 1996).

Despite these constraints, those PCGs and PCTs with a genuine commitment to developing a culture of involvement in primary care need to work out how this can extend beyond their immediate developmental and planning interests, to encompass both the quality of clinician–patient relationships and the breadth of their strategic policy concerns. *The NHS Plan* may help, both in the closer contractual relationships planned for GPs and in the potential for PCTs to 'earn' greater autonomy from the centre (Secretary of State, 2000).

## National guidance

One aspect of national policy that has not historically been overly prescriptive is, ironically, public involvement. *The NHS Plan* has specified more clearly than ever before a set of mechanisms for local public involvement, including patient forums for trusts and health authorities, and the new Patient Advocacy and Liaison Service. However, these new mechanisms do not amount to a systematic framework for public involvement. Unlike the issue of quality, which now enjoys such a framework in A *First Class Service* (Secretary of State, 1998), public involvement is still promoted as a corporate value without the detail (or the sanctions) of a plan for effective implementation.

For PCGs, lay and public involvement responsibilities have included few precise requirements and many general expectations. The former centre on having open board meetings and appointing a lay member to the board. The latter include the following:

- *[To] allow the public to participate in decisions on primary, community and hospital services* (HSC, 1998/65).
- *As Primary Care Groups are to be formed around natural geographical communities it is important that the views of local people are properly taken into account* (HSC, 1998/65).
- *Improving the health of, and addressing inequalities in, their community through ... the involvement of the public in the work of the Group so as to inform the delivery of appropriate services* (HSC, 1998/139).
- *[PCGs] will need to utilise public health skills to ensure that services are based on evidence of clinical- and cost-effectiveness, reflect users' views and an optimal balance of health service provision exists between primary,*

*community and secondary care services. For example, in commissioning hospital care for diabetes it is essential to involve patients, carers and voluntary organisations as well as clinicians* (HSC, 1998/228).

In *Patient and public involvement in the new NHS*, the NHSE made clear that public involvement was not the job of PCG lay members but had to be a corporate responsibility (Department of Health, 1999a). However, the specification of this responsibility remained elusive. There was little continuity with the set of recommendations for PCGs made a year before (NHS Executive, 1998), and a new eight-point framework for assessing progress on public involvement focused entirely on organisational process issues.

Arguably, the lack of specification of what PCGs should actually do makes it possible for local members and officers to draw on local expertise and experience in ways that are appropriate for local interests. However, the PCGs that are most in need of development input could lose out. Without clearer guidelines and priorities, poor practice will all too easily go unchecked.

## The role and contribution of lay members

The role of the lay member has been poorly defined in the NHSE guidance. In the following example, two quite different roles – one executive and one non-executive – are seamlessly merged:

> *It will be important … to involve lay members on the PCG board in order to foster local opportunities for public involvement and scrutiny of strategic and operational decisions.* (HSC, 1998/139)

Lay members have had to negotiate their roles with their ostensible peers on PCG boards, producing different results in different PCGs. Some PCG boards have welcomed and valued their lay members; others have seen the lay member as a threat and sought to marginalise him or her – differences that touch on basic attitudes about the professional role and the value of partnership with patients and lay people. Single lay members may not have had much power relative to the professional majorities on PCG boards, but their presence has forced other members to demonstrate the value they attach to lay voices. Without lay members, there would have been little to leaven the domination of professional priorities.

> I don't think I have got as much to say as some of the others but, yes, I think I am respected for the position that I am there for and I don't have any trouble. It seems to be a fairly well-gelled group: everybody is happy to talk to everybody else in the main. There is a bit of prickliness but then, you know, that is bound to happen in that the doctors know each other from BMA meetings, the nurses know each other because they both work out of the same office, and I think there is probably a dividing line between doctors and everybody else – but it is not a very obvious one. It's not, 'Oh, I won't speak to them because they're only a lay member.' You can see that people generate towards each other, but then I think that is natural and it doesn't worry me. I'm not frightened to talk to anyone.
>
> lay member

A key issue for every lay member has been defining and achieving a balance between individual contribution, as a lay person, with the promotion of other methods of lay, user and public involvement. Even where the latter task is widely acknowledged to be a corporate responsibility, lay members have typically played a key role in ensuring that public involvement stays on the PCG agenda. This has variously meant acting as a champion or advocate for public involvement work; reminding the other members of their responsibilities to consider the interests of users and their local population; leading specific initiatives; and, not least, actually going out and doing the work.

In London, very few PCG boards have left the lay member with sole responsibility for public involvement. There was almost always at least one other board member and/or a subgroup to support the work. Yet without the lay members, there can be little doubt that PCGs' public involvement ambitions would have been much slighter. Single lay members may not be able to represent their communities, but they have helped to ensure that PCG boards take the interests of local people seriously.

## Resources

The obstacles to public involvement in PCGs have been dominated not by cultural resistance but by the more mundane and familiar issue of organisational capacity. Three-quarters of the PCG chief executives in London claimed that developing public involvement was a high personal priority. But they had many 'high priorities' and, in relative terms, public involvement slipped to the lower end of their commitments. They simply have too much to do. Lack of time and resources, and the demands of the development agenda, were identified as obstacles by three-quarters of both chief executives and lay members. A recent study of practice level involvement work reported similar findings (Brown, 2000).

This is a crucial issue for the future of public involvement work. The enthusiasm of so many of the new leaders in primary care for public involvement is a real opportunity for change, but if this enthusiasm is not appropriately supported, initiatives will continue to struggle. Motivation must be accompanied by investment in time, skills and infrastructure (Porter and Coupe, 1997).

Public involvement should not, however, be seen solely as a demand on resources. A long-term vision should embrace public involvement as a route to enhancing the resources of PCGs. Building partnerships with local community stakeholders takes time and effort, but it delivers a much greater capacity for the long-term participation of local people in PCG interests.

Community Health Councils (CHCs) have long had a formal role in promoting the interests of health service users, and in many places they have become partners in developing involvement initiatives as well as contributing, as observers, at board level. Their loss will, in some places, have a significant impact on PCG public involvement work. The voluntary and community sector also offers a wealth of possibilities to PCGs seeking support through partnership, although the capacity of the voluntary sector to provide this support remains a perennial problem. Although in many areas there is little history of primary care professionals working collaboratively with such community stakeholders, the change of focus of PCG responsibilities from practice lists to the health of the local population requires that such partnerships be built.

# The nature of the task

The term 'public involvement' masks a multitude of possibilities. These have been described in the literature in various ways. The most widely used descriptive tool has been Arnstein's ladder of participation, which moves from information-giving through consultation and partnership to lay control (Arnstein, 1969). In practice, the power relationships between professionals and lay people are rarely articulated explicitly. Nonetheless, realism about the level of involvement the public can expect from statutory bodies is crucial if patients and local people are not to feel let down by the process.

Similar problems emerge in defining the aims of public involvement initiatives. Every guide to public involvement impresses upon its readers the need to be clear about aims and objectives. Yet, in practice, such a rational approach can be elusive. People join local debates about public involvement from different places, with different values and different commitments. Furthermore, the distinction between process and outcomes in public involvement work is not clear: for some, a successful public meeting may be outcome enough; for others, this is merely part of the process of delivering change for the PCG, its constituents, or for patients themselves. In such circumstances, precise definitions about outcomes can be difficult to achieve. PCG discussions on public involvement tend to be sustained by a number of different, but not necessarily conflicting, ideas about what the work is for and what may be achieved through it. All of the following aims may be embraced within such discussions, and each aim may itself be shaped by different ideas and values.

## Informing PCG decision-making and planning

This is much the most common aim identified for public involvement by PCG chief executives and lay members and, as suggested above, reflects both the nature of PCGs' responsibilities and the constraints of their position in local health economies.

## Making services more sensitive to the needs (and wants) of users

There are two characteristically different ways in which this aim is articulated. An emphasis on needs may reflect a desire for high quality needs assessment and efficient delivery of services to meet these needs. An emphasis on wants may be driven by a more consumerist agenda – the patient-centred service designed around the lives of users. Although these starting points are different, their aims are structurally very similar.

## Improving access to, and appropriate use of, primary care services

This aim encompasses the drive for equity and demand management – arguably two sides of the same coin. Those who are eager to inform local people about how to access primary care services increasingly have to attend to the concerns of other professionals in PHCTs, whose concerns are more focused on educating people about *when* to use primary care services.

## Monitoring and improving performance and standards of delivery

Users of services have an obvious role to play in ensuring the quality of those services. Although this is recognised within PCGs, their distance from the actual delivery of services has meant that this aim has not been given the priority it deserves. User involvement in clinical governance is not common (Wilkin *et al.* 2000).

## Educating local people about their health

The contribution of public involvement to public health goals is conceived both as a traditional exercise in education and as a more participative process in which engagement is a necessary precursor to education about health. In both cases, the existence of pre-determined public health education priorities is assumed.

## Empowering local people to gain control over their health and health care

Although similar to the last aim, this is a more radical vision rooted in the principles of community development rather than public health (although there is a long-established overlap between the two). The emphasis here is on enabling people to identify and address their own health needs, rather than imposing professional solutions. However, this aim operates at the individual level as well as at the community level, informed by a desire to promote self-care and personal autonomy in managing health issues.

## Building partnerships with local communities

As suggested above, partnership with local communities may reasonably be perceived as a crucial goal in itself. This may be informed by a belief in the value of civil society or simply by a need to be sensitive to local politics.

## Encouraging accountable and open processes

Openness is a relatively simple principle of good public governance that the Government has promoted in the health service, despite its evident anxieties elsewhere (e.g. the emasculated Freedom of Information Bill). But the broader issues of accountability remain fraught within the health service. The new NHS Appointments Commission will improve the appointment of non-executive directors, but the system as a whole remains weak.

Given the diversity of these aims and the multiplicity of world-views and political values that underpin them, it is hardly surprising that PCGs have not been rigorous in defining what they want to achieve through public involvement. Greater clarity is needed, but achieving this clarity will require skill in identifying and acknowledging the interests of all local stakeholders. In practice, PCGs are likely to find themselves pursuing approaches to involvement that draw on both consumerist and democratic visions of what the process is about. Activity will change over time to reflect different purposes, ideologies and audiences (Brown, 2000).

*Our lay member comes from the voluntary sector and they have huge amounts of experience – far more than we do in the health service – of engaging people meaningfully on issues. They are motivated; they're not just passing through, seeing the GP with a snotty nose, you know. So she gets a bit impatient with it all and I have a lot of sympathy for her, but I do think this is a tough area because we are culturally diverse as a group and we're all coming at it from different angles and so it's a really huge challenge. I think she gets a bit fed up with it all really because she sees the power, the hierarchy, as being almost impenetrable, you know – how do you ever challenge that power base of GP and patient?*

PCG officer

## The future of public involvement in Primary Care Groups and Trusts

For all the enthusiasm of the new advocates for public involvement in primary care, PCGs – like other NHS institutions – remain structurally insensitive to patient and public views. Interest in the methods of public involvement is not matched by attention to the internal processes whereby learning from public involvement initiatives turns into changes in policy and practice. It is widely assumed that there are implicit mechanisms for achieving this, when in fact the opposite is the case: the mechanisms within the health service for responding to patient and public voices are very weak indeed. The power of the professionals and the institutions is ingrained. There is a constant risk that professionals will sign up to the rhetoric of public involvement but do no more than manipulate the process to legitimate their own decisions and interests (Harrison and Mort, 1998). Despite being described as participants, patients and members of the public remain observers without real access to the decision arena: while being in the game, they are more reserves than players (Brownlea, 1987).

In the foreseeable future, this state of affairs is unlikely to change radically. *The NHS Plan* claims a vision of a 'health service designed around the patient', but its content does not take this vision seriously – or rather it constructs the 'patient' as a consumer, not as an individual with rights, values, ideas, interests, commitments and knowledge. To value everything that patients and local people can bring to the development of health services will require more far-reaching change in both the institutions and the professions. It is too early to say what benefits or otherwise the new mechanisms in *The NHS Plan* will bring. In practice, this will depend on how the bones are fleshed out in meaningful local processes.

In the meantime, the major developmental challenge facing most PCGs is the move to PCT status. This change turns (relatively small) primary care development organisations into (often larger) serious NHS institutions: the full weight of corporate governance descends and the experimental PCG boards are replaced by 'proper' NHS trust boards with executive committees beneath them. Lay members disappear in the process, although many will no doubt become part of the new non-executive majorities on PCT boards. The implications of these changes for the public involvement agenda are ambiguous – there are both threats and opportunities inherent in the process.

The greatest threat in the short term may simply lie in the turmoil of yet more change. The gains that have been made are likely to be fragile and so may be easily swept away, especially when mergers are involved. Organisational change also undermines the development of trust in individual and organisational partnerships. This impact is most damaging where those partnerships are weakest. The common perception that the health service is always in the process of change is a major disincentive to active engagement with it. PCGs must therefore ensure some degree of continuity in these partnerships, even if this is only at officer level, in order that they do not have to be built again from scratch.

However, PCT development offers an opportunity to build on what has been learned and to establish more thorough-going processes of involvement in organisational process. A PCT ought to be the fruition of the PCG developmental process: turning the learning and experience of the new primary care corporacy into mature institutional expression. Where there has been real enthusiasm in PCGs for public involvement, this ought to be reflected in the commitments and priorities of their emergent PCT boards.

*The most important part is us going out and listening, but you then have to do something with what you're heard. You can't just take it in and hold onto it – the point of doing listening is to actually feedback through to somewhere. At the moment, the mechanisms for that just aren't clearly established.*

*I think the way we do the PCT consultation and how we take forward the lessons we have learned in the PCG about sharing good practice and about what works well and what doesn't work well – these things should inform the community involvement strategy that the PCT then adopts.*

PCG officer

Whatever their inheritance, PCTs cannot ignore their patient and public involvement responsibilities. In the NHSE guidance on establishing PCTs, public involvement was identified as one of four key principles underpinning their governance arrangements (Department of Health, 1999b):

*PCTs need to be firmly rooted in the local community and be responsive to local people's health needs and wishes. This calls for the direct involvement of lay people drawn from the local community (including local government): it also calls for continuing dialogue with various stakeholders in the local community over the planning and delivery of services.*

In the detailed corporate governance framework produced for PCTs prior to the first wave going live in April 2000, six key functions were identified for PCT boards for which they are held accountable by the NHS Executive on behalf of the Secretary of State (NHS Executive, 2000). The sixth is:

*to ensure that the Executive Committee leads an effective dialogue between the organisation and the local community on its plans and performance and that these are responsive to the community's needs.*

This explicit statement of the duties of the Executive Committee, linked to the critical scrutiny of the board, ought to place public involvement squarely at the centre of PCT officers' concerns. Whether this is achieved will depend on many factors, not least the interests, priorities and capacity of the officers, and the determination and commitment of the board members to see this function realised.

Where lay members have played an important role in advocating or doing public involvement (the majority of PCGs), their loss may have important consequences that PCG officers should anticipate. The non-executive role is a different role, with its own history in the health service. Although it embraces accountability to the local community, its focus is on governance and scrutiny. The PCT governance framework makes clear that although non-executives should bring their wider experience to bear on the concerns of the PCT, their attitude should be one of 'critical detachment'. The business of actually 'doing' public involvement is, as with all PCT business, left to the Executive Board.

The outlook is not discouraging. Patient and public involvement in primary care is now supported by both formal commitments within organisational governance arrangements and the considerable personal commitments of many of the officers and members responsible for taking primary care development forward. We may be a long way from a service that genuinely treats its patients and public as partners, but those who promote this ideal are no longer voices in the wilderness.

## References

Allen P. Clinical governance in primary care: Accountability for clinical governance: developing collective responsibility for quality in primary care. BMJ 2000; 321: 608–11.

Anderson W, Florin D. Involving the public – one of many priorities. London: King's Fund, 2000.

Arnstein S R. A ladder of citizen partnership, Journal of the American Planning Association 1969; 35 (4): 216–24.

Barnes M, McIver S. Public Participation in Primary Care. Birmingham: University of Birmingham Health Service Management Centre, 1999.

Brown I. Community and participation for general practice: perceptions of general practitioners and community nurses. Social Science and Medicine 1994; 39 (3): 335–44.

Brown I. Involving the public in general practice in an urban district: levels and type of activity and perceptions of obstacles. Health and Social Care in the Community 2000; 8 (4): 251–59.

Brownlea A. Participation: myths, realities and prognosis. Social Science and Medicine 1987; 25 (6): 605–14.

Department of Health. *Patient and public involvement in the new NHS*. London: Department of Health, 1999a.

Department of Health. *Primary Care Trusts. Establishing Better Services*. London: Department of Health, 1999b.

Fisher B, Neve H, Heritage Z. Community development, user involvement, and primary health care. *BMJ* 1999; 318: 749–50.

Harrison S, Mort M. Which champions, which people? Public and user involvement in health care as a technology of legitimation. *Social Policy & Administration* 1998; 32 (1): 60–70.

Huntington J, Gillam S, Rosen R. Clinical governance in primary care: Organisational development for clinical governance. *BMJ* 2000; 321: 679–82.

NHS Executive, IHSM, NHS Confederation. *In the Public Interest: Developing a Strategy for Public Participation in the NHS*. London: Department of Health, 1998.

NHS Executive. *PCT corporate governance framework*. Leeds: NHS Executive, 2000.

Porter S, Coupe M. What happens to local voices in a primary care led NHS? *British Journal of Health Care Management* 1997; 3 (10): 533–35.

Rogers A, Popay J. User involvement in primary care. In: *What is the Future for a Primary Care-led NHS?* University of Manchester National Primary Care Research and Development Centre, editor. Oxford: Radcliffe Medical Press, 1997: 13–19.

Secretary of State for Health. *The New NHS: modern, dependable*. London: Department of Health, 1997.

Secretary of State for Health. *A First Class Service*. London: Department of Health, 1998.

Secretary of State for Health. *The NHS Plan*. London: Department of Health, 2000.

Wilkin D, Gillam S, Leese B. *The National Tracker Survey of Primary Care Groups and Trusts. Progress and Challenges 1999/2000*. Manchester: The University of Manchester, 2000.

Winkler F. Involving patients. In: Meads G, editor. *A Primary Care-led NHS*. London: Churchill Livingstone, 1996: 117–29.

Chapter 4

# Partnership in the primary care consultation

Dominique Florin and Angela Coulter

## KEY POINTS

- An understanding of the primary care consultation has evolved that incorporates a holistic view of health, a patient-centred view of medicine and a dynamic role for the doctor–patient relationship.

- There is good evidence that in most situations, patients want better communication and information in consultations, and that this leads to greater patient satisfaction and improved concordance with treatment decisions.

- The evidence that patients want to share decision-making with doctors is more equivocal, and more research is needed to elucidate which patients, in which circumstances, want and will benefit from shared decision-making.

- Health professionals need skills to guage patient preferences in different situations, and skills to share information and decision-making. There are a growing number of decision aids being developed to help with this process.

## Introduction

The primary care consultation is a key building block of the relationship between patients/users and health services. The vast majority of contacts between health services and users take place at the primary care level. Most users will never become involved in primary care policy, but sooner or later virtually all will come into contact with primary care services through a consultation. Thus, the quality and characteristics of the relationship between user and health professional in that consultation is fundamental to users' experience of health care and the extent to which it can be understood as a partnership. In this chapter, we will consider some of the ways in which users and professionals interact at the level of the primary care consultation, in particular the trend to greater involvement of patients in decisions about their care. The chapter has a tripartite structure – we consider, in turn, the evolving nature of the primary care consultation, power and partnership in the relationship between doctors and patients, and finally shared decision-making, an area that has recently become more prominent.

## Ways of conceiving primary care and the consultation

In the last 50 years, a variety of models have been elaborated that allow us to understand primary care and the consultation in different ways. Essentially these models are based on different understandings of health, of the function of medical care, and of the aims of the consultation. Two such models are shown in Table 4.1 below. The point about this type of work is that there are many different ways of describing the world of general practice and the consultation, which are not necessarily mutually exclusive.

**Table 4.1** Models of general practice

| Pendleton et al. (1984) | Toon (1994) |
| --- | --- |
| medical | biomedical |
| sociological | holistic/psychoanalytic |
| anthropological | preventive |
| psychological | entrepreneurial |

In relation to patient participation, two particular models are of interest. The first is the biomedical model, often seen as the classical or traditional approach to medical practice. Crudely put, this places biomedical knowledge at the centre of the consultation: knowledge controlled by a paternalistic doctor and meted out in the form of management decisions to a passive patient. In opposition there are a number of 'patient-centred' models of practice, which to varying degrees recognise the importance of patients' own views in determining the course of the consultation and future encounters. To some extent this is a false dichotomy, for these two apparently conflicting models can and do co-exist, even within the gamut of approaches used by a single practitioner with respect to a single patient. One of the challenges in this area is to determine the circumstances in which different models of consultation are appropriate.

## The development of patient-centred medicine

One of the earliest and most influential exponents of patient-centred medicine was the psychotherapist Michael Balint (1957). Whilst part of Balint's approach is about putting patients' views at the centre of the consultation, other components include the use of the doctor–patient relationship as a therapeutic tool, and the importance of the doctor's self-awareness of his or her own life experiences. Since this early work, many others have added to the patient-centred model of medicine, a few of which are mentioned here.

The work of Pendleton (1984) and colleagues emphasised the need for doctors to elicit the triad of patients' ideas, concerns and expectations in order to achieve a satisfactory outcome in the consultation. Stewart *et al.* (1995) developed the notion of the patient in partnership with health professionals and implied a change in the balance of power between doctors and patients. Most recently, work by Elwyn, Edwards and Kinnersley (1999) and Gwyn and Elwyn (1999) has moved the agenda on by focusing on the 'neglected second half of the consultation'. This is an important progression, which clarifies the need not just to be sensitive to the patient's (not always explicit) agenda in order to accurately characterise the problem, but also to work with the patient in order to achieve a shared solution.

Despite the fact that it is possible to distinguish a historical trend towards patient-centred medicine, we do not really know how prevalent it is. We know from the work of Byrne and Long (1976) that at that time doctor-centred consultations were common, but we have little evidence as to the extent to which this has changed. Recent work by Elwyn, Edwards, Gwyn and Grol (1999) with general practice trainees suggests that there is some way to go before partnership in the second half of the consultation is achieved. The sharing of information is more accepted by clinicians than sharing decision-making, and in many cases by patients also (McKinstry, 2000). At the same time, work by authors such as Pendleton *et al.* has widely influenced GP training.

## Aims and outcomes of the consultation

One common feature of the approaches described above is that they are based on a holistic view of health. Health states reflect not only biomedical attributes but also social and psychological factors. Indeed, these may be the more important and require doctors to develop methods of working with patients that extend beyond the traditional biomedical model.

One difficulty is that there is no universal agreement as to what should be the aim or outcome of a consultation in primary care. This is a fundamental problem. As Toon has pointed out, part of the difficulty in measuring quality in general practice stems from a lack of consensus as to what general practice is for. There are several possible goals of a primary care consultation (see Table 4.2).

**Table 4.2** Possible goals of primary care consultations

- patient satisfaction
- patient enablement
- compliance with treatment
- improved biomedical status
- improved well-being
- health understanding
- cost-effective resource use
- public health benefit (as in screening or immunisation)

Whilst the ideal might be for all these outcomes to co-exist, in reality they sometimes conflict. Austoker (1999) has pointed out that the public health gain of a screening programme may be in conflict with the patient's choice not to take part. Coulter (1999) suggests that, even where increased patient choice results in greater health expenditure, this may be a worthwhile outcome. However, there is no consensus on this view. From both a pragmatic and a research point of view, the lack of a single or simple measure of outcome in primary care raises a question about the aim of patient-centred medicine: is patient enablement an aim in its own right or is it a means to another outcome such as improved compliance? A holistic view of health implies that a satisfactory outcome must extend beyond measurable biomedical improvement to include social and emotional factors. Only an approach that recognises all these components will achieve both health improvement and patient satisfaction.

## Organisational aspects affecting the nature of the consultation and the partnership between patient and professional

Traditionally a consultation takes place in the context of a relationship between a patient and his or her usual doctor or GP. However, recent developments in the organisation of primary care revise this understanding. Increasingly, patients are registered with large group practices that do not operate personal list systems. This makes continuity of care with a particular GP less likely. We know relatively little about the impact of continuity on patient partnership and choice, but the evidence suggests that most patients do value continuity though this may be traded off against ease of access (Guthrie and Wyke, 2000).

An increasing number of consultations take place with a nurse rather than a doctor, whether for minor illnesses or chronic conditions. Patient satisfaction with nurse consultations is often high, and some research has shown that nurses provide information more effectively than doctors do (Iliffe, 2000), but little is known about whether continuity or a participative style are key factors in patients' responses to nurse consultations. The advent of nurse-led telephone helplines such as NHS Direct and nurse-led walk-in centres herald a new form of access to health advice in which on-going relationships are unlikely to be a feature. These services allow patients direct access to nurse consultations over the phone or face to face and are often led by a computer-generated protocol. The style is likely to be directive advice-giving rather than information-sharing and preference elicitation.

In comparison with many other Western countries, the NHS is a 'low choice' system. Patients must be registered and consult with only one practice; they cannot consult with several GPs simultaneously. There is no open access to specialists or secondary care. The lack of a direct financial relationship between doctor and patient is also at variance with the situation in some other systems. Reforms in the 1980s and 1990s were presented as increasing the customer aspect of the patient's role, but it is not clear that this was achieved. What impact do these organisational factors have on the relationship between doctor and patient? There is some work on international comparisons which suggests that hospital patients in the UK are particularly unlikely to feel involved in health care decisions. We do not fully understand the reasons for these differences. Most of the literature on patient partnership and shared decision-making has looked at the dynamics and events within the consultation, rather than at the organisational or financial setting within which the consultation is held.

## Power, paternalism and partnership – relationships between users and professionals

McWhinney (1995) states that although patient-centred medicine does improve patients' health, this is not its prime aim. Rather, its aim is a moral one: to redress the imbalance of power that has become inherent in modern medicine. Certainly the redistribution of power in the doctor–patient relationship has come to be seen as the basis of the patient-centred medicine movement.

A recent important development has been the notion of the 'patient as expert', particularly in the case of chronic diseases. At its basis is the conviction that only a person who is experiencing a specific condition really knows what it is like, particularly with respect to areas other than the strictly biomedical, such as emotional and social aspects. With a holistic view of health all these factors contribute to health and well-being, and it is thus crucial to take account of them in assessing treatment choices. Because only the patient has access to some of these areas of information, it follows that the patient must be the ultimate arbiter of what will improve his or her health. The work described by Gilbert and Fisher later in this book tests the limits of this in relation to clinical effectiveness.

### Power in the consultation

What are the sources of professional power in the medical consultation? Pendleton *et al.* (1984) present a tripartite classification shown in Table 4.3 overleaf.

**Table 4.3** Sources of power in the consultation    Pendleton *et al.* (1984)

- power based on knowledge
- power based on the moral authority to do good for patients
- 'charismatic authority' based on the aspect of healing that stems from the conjunction of medicine with mystery and religion

The first two forms of power are more straightforwardly related to the subject under discussion. Clearly, knowledge is a central component of the consultation, and health professionals are the repository of much clinical knowledge. However, as pointed out above, there are some areas of knowledge to which only the patient can have access. Much previously inaccessible technical information is now available to patients, for example through the Internet. Thus, power based on knowledge is not confined to health professionals. The same applies to the second type of power, based on the motive to do good, or 'beneficence' in ethical terms. If the patient is the expert with respect to his or her own experience of illness, it cannot be the case that the doctor alone decides what is good for the patient. Silverman (1987) illustrates the third, more complex, type of authority with the suggestion that power imbalance in the consultation may be necessary for a variety of reasons, including that it is in some sense linked to patients' belief in health professionals' healing powers. As a practical example, Silverman quotes the case of parents of a child with Down's Syndrome for whom cardiac surgery is being considered. The parents' reluctance to make a choice that could lead to their child's death, and thus their choice to leave responsibility for the treatment decision to the doctor, is given as an example of the necessary power imbalance in the consultation. As will be discussed below, this is an example where a paternalistic approach is appropriate but where a sufficiently open communication style is needed to elicit this preference.

## Partnership and shared decision-making in the consultation

As we have said above, there are many possible outcomes of a primary care consultation. Not all of these involve decision-making; for example where the doctor simply listens to the patient's account of a particular experience. Even where there is no overt decision-making, there is still scope for partnership. The dictionary definition of 'partnership' implies a joint undertaking or shared enterprise, and the underlying attributes must be that each contributor is held in equal value and that there is good communication, verbal or otherwise. Unfortunately, this is by no means the universal experience in primary care. Both doctors and patients may be difficult, and failures in communication are common (Barry *et al.* 2000; Britten *et al.* 2000). The organisational changes described above, which impact on continuity of care, may also compromise partnership. In addition, most GP consultations are only ten minutes long or less, and we know from Howie *et al.*'s work (1997) that patient enablement is related to consultation length. Lack of time is also frequently quoted as a barrier to patient-centred medicine and shared decision-making, although training, decision aids and attitudinal change may counteract this to some extent (Coulter, 1997; Stewart *et al.* 1995). Dissatisfaction with communication in the consultation is suggested by evidence showing that some groups, particularly younger and non-White patients, tend to feel that they receive insufficient information from their doctors (National Health Service Executive, 1999). (Chapter 6 illustrates how an appreciation of minority ethnic health beliefs can enhance information exchange in the management of asthma.)

## The spectrum from paternalism to consumer choice

One area of the consultation that has recently received attention is that of decision-making around treatment options. It has been suggested that this mainly concerns patients with serious and chronic diseases (Towle and Godolphin, 1999), but decisions are also frequently made for relatively trivial acute complaints such as the management of viral infections, which can, nevertheless, set the tone of the continuing relationship. What is needed is an approach that encompasses all these situations. Decision-making is an area of the consultation that has been subject to a growing body of research. A spectrum of approaches has been developed, as outlined in Table 4.4 below.

**Table 4.4** Approaches to decision-making in the consultation

- paternalism
- shared decision-making
- consumer choice

At the most 'doctor-led' end is traditional paternalism, where the doctor owns and manages all the information and decides on the patient's behalf what the management should be. The disadvantages of this model have been rehearsed above, but there are times when it is the patient's preferred approach. In a critical acute situation, for example suffering a heart attack, it may be the most appropriate course of action.

At the other end of the spectrum is consumer choice, whereby the doctor's principal role is to present all available information to the patient and then allow the patient a free choice in deciding any treatment option. Clearly in this approach information is fully shared, but power regarding treatment choice is entirely delegated to the patient. This approach implies a high level of patient autonomy but may not always produce individual or public health benefits. It may also leave the patient feeling anxious and abandoned (Elwyn, Edwards and Kinnersley, 1999).

Between these two extremes, though also qualitatively different, lies shared decision-making. This model incorporates pure information-sharing with a shared approach to decision-making that involves both patient and doctor. Shared decision-making is qualitatively different from the other two models because it explicitly gives a role to the relationship between the doctor and the patient, and in this respect owes a debt to the Balint approach. It is also the most dynamic of the models, with the possibility of varying the balance of power and information according to circumstance. It recognises the dynamic nature of decision-making in the consultation (Charles, Gafni and Whelan, 2000).

In shared decision-making, patients and health professionals share both the process of decision-making and ownership of the decision made. Shared information about values and likely treatment outcomes is an essential prerequisite, but the process also depends on a commitment from both parties to engage in a negotiated decision-making process. The clinician has to be prepared to acknowledge the legitimacy of the patient's preferences and the patient has to accept shared responsibility for the treatment decision.

## Consequences of sharing information and decisions

As was stated in the introduction to this book, there is much evidence as to the benefits of improved communication and shared information between doctors and patients. We know that patients generally, though not always, want more information than they get (Hope, 1996; Coulter, Entwistle and Gilbert, 1998; National Health Service Executive, 1999). We know also that doctors frequently underestimate how much information patients want (Strull *et al.* 1984), and that doctors may often be unaware of their patients' preferences (Coulter *et al.* 1994). However, because patients do not always want more information, doctors need specific skills to elicit patient preferences on information-sharing. There is also a body of evidence which suggests that outcomes such as patient satisfaction, health status and compliance with treatment decisions are better when patients are well-informed (Greenfield *et al.* 1988; Hope, 1996; Coulter, 1997; McKinstry, 2000).

Less is known, however, about the extent to which patients want to share decisions rather than just information. This is an important distinction. A number of studies have investigated the extent of desire for participation among different groups of patients (Cassileth *et al.* 1980; Anell *et al.* 1997; Stiggelbout *et al.* 1997). Desire for participation varies according to age, educational status, disease group and cultural background. The age differences in decision-making preferences suggest that the preference for active involvement may be increasing over time, reflecting greater knowledge of the risks as well as the benefits of medical care, and decreased willingness to submit to the authority of clinicians.

Some patients in certain situations undoubtedly prefer a directive, doctor-led style (Savage, 1990; McKinstry, 2000). Health professionals need to regularly re-assess the appropriate approach in relation to any particular patient. This point is illustrated in work by Degner and Sloan (1992), which shows that whilst most healthy patients stated that should they develop cancer they would wish to select their own treatment, many patients with cancer did not share this view. For a doctor to adopt a decision-sharing approach, where this is not what the patient wants, this could have a negative impact, increasing uncertainty and anxiety.

## Decision aids

From the preceding section, it is clear that shared decision-making requires health professionals to use a sophisticated range of skills both to elicit patient preferences and then actually to share information and decisions as appropriate. This is a daunting task in the face of a busy and demanding clinical case-load. A frequent objection to shared decision-making has been that it requires far more time than is currently available in routine general practice. Authors are divided on this issue. Some suggest that a patient-centred style of consulting and shared decision-making is possible within a ten-minute consultation (Towle and Godolphin, 1999); others acknowledge that more time is needed (McKinstry, 2000).

One approach being developed that will address some of the time and resource concerns is the use of decision aids. An important part of the patient-centred agenda requires the communication to patients of technical data, often including complex risk assessments that incorporate individual characteristics. This does not necessarily need to take place with a health professional present, thus easing time and resource constraints. Decision aids are useful in conditions where there are several management options, whether for screening, diagnosis or treatment. They may involve individual or group interview, written material, graphic representations, audio-visual or computer simulations. They may be interactive to incorporate patients' questions and preferences. Most proponents of shared decision-making argue that it is important to ensure that the patient has access to unbiased, evidence-based information where it exists, and information about knowledge gaps and uncertainties wherever relevant (Hope, 1996). They must also be helped to articulate their values. This is usually done using interactive methods, sometimes involving explicit decision-analytic techniques (Feldman-Stewart et al. 2000).

Decision aids improve knowledge, reduce uncertainty and decisional conflict, do not increase anxiety, and stimulate active involvement (O'Connor et al. 1999). They have been shown to affect treatment choices, but whether they increase satisfaction or result in improved health outcomes is still a matter for debate (O'Connor et al. 1999; Edwards and Elwyn, 1999; Man-Son-Hing et al. 1999).

Determining which outcomes are important in the evaluation of a patient decision aid takes us back to the problem of the purpose of the consultation and the reasons why the decision aid was developed in the first place. Patient involvement in health care decision-making has been encouraged for a variety of reasons and can be justified with reference to different theoretical frameworks (Entwistle *et al.* 1998).

From an ethical standpoint, the main rationale may be to support patients' autonomy or self-determination. If patients are to be supported in autonomous decision-making, they require good quality, evidence-based information about treatment options and their relative effectiveness so that they can make informed choices. In this case the outcome of interest may be the extent to which patients feel sufficiently informed and confident to make autonomous decisions. Involvement in decision-making is the key aim of the intervention, but the actual nature of the decisions or choices made will be of less interest.

A variant on this approach would also focus on the process of decision-making rather than the outcome, but would see the achievement of concordance with the patient's preferred decision-making style as of greatest interest. So patients who do not want to be actively involved in making treatment choices should not be pressurised to do so. From this perspective, achieving a high level of involvement is less important than the patient's satisfaction with the decision-making process. A 'good' decision is one in which both the patient's preferred level of involvement and his/her values and preferences are explicitly incorporated into the treatment choice.

An alternative approach would place more stress on the consequences of patient involvement in decision-making measured in terms of the choices made and the effects on these choices. For example, those concerned to secure more effective use of health service resources might look for evidence that care given was more appropriate and better tailored to patients' needs as a result of involving them in decision-making. From this perspective, improvements in health status might be the outcome of primary interest.

Others might hope that greater knowledge and empowerment of patients would lead to more efficient use of health care resources. They would therefore be interested in finding out whether the intervention reduced demand for expensive or risky procedures and increased the likelihood that patients would feel able to care for themselves without recourse to medical interventions.

Unfortunately, few patient information materials currently in use in the NHS have been designed to support decision-making. On the contrary, a recent review found that most patient leaflets and videos were of poor quality, containing inaccurate, out-of-date, biased and unreliable information (Coulter, Entwistle and Gilbert, 1998). The potential benefit of decision aids will not be realised unless these problems are resolved.

## Training issues

Despite the growing panoply of decision aids described above, their use requires not just technical training but also changes in attitudes. One barrier to implementation is that shared decision-making requires specific skills that are not yet widely taught. Elwyn, Edwards and Kinnersley (1999) have demonstrated that new skills are needed to move from the well-established Pendleton agenda of uncovering patients' 'ideas, concerns and expectations', to a position where genuine shared decision-making is possible. This requires rigorous attention to later stages of the clinical encounter.

Further, GP registrars have demonstrated practitioners' reluctance to take on a patient-centred approach in the second half of the consultation, despite their stated adherence to these principles at the stage of defining the agenda (Elwyn et al. 1999). Part of the difficulty lies in doctors' attitudes and reluctance to relinquish power or to reveal the true level of uncertainty that often exists in clinical decision-making. The clinician also has to deal with the difficulty of establishing what level of decision-sharing is appropriate in any given circumstance, and then modifying his or her approach in consequence. Towle and Godolphin (1999) have attempted to define the competencies required by doctors for shared decision-making, including such areas as identifying choices, presenting evidence and negotiating decisions in partnership. Many of these competencies should already be in the gamut of skills taught to doctors in training, but what is required is an attitudinal change to use these skills systematically, with the aim of sharing not just information but also decisions. Towle and Godolphin have also begun to identify patient competencies required, including developing a partnership relationship with a doctor and evaluating evidence. The approach demonstrates the degree to which patients need to be explicitly and actively involved in the process of shared decision-making. We do not yet know how willing and able patients will be to engage with this demanding agenda (Gambrill, 1999).

# References

Anell A, Rosen P, Hjortsberg C. Choice and participation in the health services: a survey of preferences among Swedish residents. *Health Policy* 1997; 40: 157–68.

Austoker J. Gaining informed consent for screening. *BMJ* 1999; 319: 722.

Balint M. *The Doctor, his Patient and the Illness.* London: Pitman, 1957.

Barry *et al.* Patients' unvoiced agendas in general practice consultations: qualitative study. *BMJ* 2000; 320: 1246–50.

Britten *et al.* Misunderstandings in prescribing decisions in general practice: qualitative study. *BMJ* 2000; 320: 484–88.

Byrne P, Long B. *Doctors talking to patients.* London: DHSS, 1980.

Cassileth B R, Zupkis R V, Sutton-Smith K, March V. Information and participation preferences of hospitalised adult cancer patients. *Annals of Internal Medicine* 1980; 92: 832.

Charles C, Gafni A, Whelan T. How to improve communication between doctors and patients. *BMJ* 2000; 320: 1220–21.

Coulter A, Peto V, Doll H. Patients' preferences and general practitioners' decisions in the treatment of menstrual disorders. *Family Practice* 1994; 11: 67–74.

Coulter A. Partnerships with patients: the pros and cons of shared clinical decision-making. *Journal of Health Services Research* 1997; 2: 112–21.

Coulter A, Entwistle V, Gilbert D. *Informing patients.* London: King's Fund, 1998.

Coulter A. Paternalism or partnership? *BMJ* 1999; 319: 719.

Degner L, Sloan J. Decision making during serious illness: what role do patients really want to play? *Journal of Clinical Epidemiology* 1992; 45: 941–50.

Edwards A, Elwyn G. The Potential benefits of Decision Aids in Clinical Medicine. *Journal of the American Medical Association* 1999; 282: 779–80.

Elwyn G, Edwards A, Kinnersley P. Shared decision-making in primary care: the neglected second half of the consultation. *British Journal of General Practice* 1999; 49: 477–82.

Elwyn G, Edwards A, Gwyn R, Grol R. Towards a feasible model for shared decision making: focus group study with general practice registrars. *BMJ* 1999; 319: 753–56.

Entwistle V A, Sowden A J, Watt I S. Evaluating interventions to promote patient involvement in decision-making: by what criteria should effectiveness be judged? *Journal of Health Services Research and Policy* 1998; 3: 100–07.

Feldman-Stewart D, Brundage M D, McConnell B A, Mackillop W J. Practical issues in assisting shared decision-making. *Health Expectations* 2000; 3: 46–54.

Gambrill J. Commentary: Proposals based on too many assumptions. *BMJ* 1999; 319: 766–71.

Greenfield S *et al*. Patients' participation in medical care: effects on blood sugar control and quality of life in diabetes. *Journal of General and Internal Medicine* 1988; 3: 448–57.

Guthrie B, Wyke S. Does continuity in general practice really matter? *BMJ* 2000; 321: 734–36.

Gwyn R, Elwyn G. When is a shared decision not (quite) a shared decision? Negotiating preferences in a general practice encounter. *Social Science and Medicine* 1999; 49: 437–47.

Hope T. *Evidence-Based Patient Choice*. London: King's Fund, 1996.

Howie J, Heaney D, Maxwell M. *Measuring quality in general practice*. RCGP Paper 75. London: Royal College of General Practitioners, 1997.

Iliffe S. Nursing and the future of primary care. *BMJ* 2000; 320: 1020–21.

Man-Son-Hing *et al*. A patient decision aid regarding anti-thrombotic therapy for stroke prevention in atrial fibrillation: a randomized controlled trial. *Journal of the American Medical Association* 1999; 282: 737–43.

McKinstry B. Do patients wish to be involved in decision making in the consultation? A cross sectional survey with video vignettes. *BMJ* 2000; 321: 867–71.

McWhinney I. Why we need a new clinical method. In: Stewart M *et al*. *Patient-Centered Medicine. Transforming the Clinical Method*. Thousand Oaks: Sage, 1995.

National Health Service Executive. *National surveys of NHS patients. General practice 1998*. London: NHSE, 1999.

O'Connor A *et al*. Decision aids for patients facing health treatment or screening decisions: systematic review. *BMJ* 1999; 319: 731–34.

Pendleton D, Schofield T, Tate P, Havelock P. *The consultation: An approach to learning and teaching*. Oxford: Oxford University Press, 1984.

Savage R. Effect of a general practitioner's consulting style on patient satisfaction: a controlled study. *BMJ* 1990; 301: 968–70.

Silverman D. *Communications and Medical Practice. Social Relations in the clinic.* London: Sage, 1987.

Stewart M *et al*. *Patient-Centered Medicine. Transforming the Clinical Method.* Thousand Oaks: Sage, 1995.

Stiggelbout A M, Kiebert G M. Patient preferences regarding information and participation in clinical decision-making. *Canadian Medical Association Journal* 1997; 157: 383–89.

Strull W, Lo B, Charles G. Do patients want to participate in medical decision making? *Journal of the American Medical Association* 1984; 252: 2990–94.

Toon P D. *What is Good General Practice? A Philosophical Study of the Concept of High Quality Medical Care.* RCGP Occasional Paper 65. London: Royal College of General Practitioners, 1994.

Towle A, Godolphin W. Framework for teaching and learning informed shared decision making. *BMJ* 1999; 319: 766–71.

# Part II

# User voices

# Introduction to the case study chapters

The following case study chapters aim to provide illustrations of the dilemmas and challenges, as well as strategies and ways forward, explored in the conceptual chapters in Part I. The chapters are based on research findings and projects that exemplify a diversity of user voices, and the place of user involvement in the delivery of effective health care. The authors and editors recognise that this text cannot comprehensively address the full range of diversity in users' voices. The chapters, in reflecting the complexity of the issues raised in Part I, have a different feel and format from each other, as they intentionally set out to address the different elements that influence user involvement in primary health care.

In the first two chapters, Brooks considers the views and experience of women, while Lomax *et al.* explore the relationship between culture, the primary health care service and the management of asthma. These chapters are concerned with understanding user views and priorities as the basis for effective shared decision-making, as well as indicating the types of relationships providers need to encourage participative user involvement in primary health care. The next three chapters – Greatley on mental health, Banks on the carers' contribution in primary care and Edwards on developing services with older people – all seek to provide practical lessons drawn from innovative projects involving these key groups of users. Finally, Fisher and Gilbert explore user involvement in community and service development.

Chapter 5

# Leading three or four lives: women and involvement in primary care

Fiona Brooks

---

**KEY POINTS**

- In a context of low social support and multiple responsibilities, women's utilisation of the primary health care service needs to be interpreted as reasoned decision-making.

- An understanding by providers of the impact of the socio-economic context of women's lives can mark a starting point for a more participative approach to the delivery of primary health care.

- Shared control over decision-making is particularly valued by women, and some evidence suggests that there is a willingness among women to share the responsibility for the outcome.

---

## Why *women* and primary health care?

*Oh, a 'heartsink patient' is the typical middle-aged woman who is in your surgery what seems like every week with one trivial thing after another.*

(comment from a GP)

*I think what I'd like to change more than anything is not the actual surgery because it is very pleasant to go into, it is the education of my GP. I'd like someone to sit down and re-educate him.*

(woman aged 46, four children, part-time teacher) [i]

Primary health care is centrally involved in a number of targeted services concerned with women's health care, cervical screening programmes,

---

[i] The occupations and other details listed are all as defined by the interviewees.

community-based maternity care, and the family planning services. Women represent an important user group for involvement in primary care and health promotion: women are the key health workers in the household – the primary agents of health socialisation, the food providers and the unpaid carers of the sick (Graham, 1993; Charles and Kerr, 1988). Moreover, women, particularly those aged 45 and over, consult their GPs more frequently than men and overall represent the largest users of the primary health care service (Kane, 1991).

At the policy level in the UK, responses to women's health care have focused broadly on reproductive health, as illustrated by the implementation of cervical and breast screening programmes and policy developments such as *Changing Childbirth* (Department of Health, 1993). Undoubtedly, these have resulted in an attempt to reduce mortality rates from cancer and in some localities a more humanised maternity service. However, the result of the focus on reproductive health has resulted in a general perception that women's needs have been dealt with (Thomas, 1996) and that it is male health that now requires attention (Lyons and Willott, 1999).

However, the notion that the major issues in women's health have been addressed is problematic. This chapter will aim to indicate that an assessment of women's needs in the construction of primary health care requires further development (Doyal, 1991). Through accounts from women and providers, the importance for women of participative approaches to the delivery of primary care will be highlighted. Finally, the chapter will illustrate how providers, particularly at the level of the consultation, can start to approach shared decision-making based on an appreciation of the socio-economic context of women's lives.

## The Women and Primary Health Care Project

The material discussed in this chapter is drawn from a study concerned with delivery of care for women by the primary care sector. The 'Women and Primary Health Care Project' (WPHC) set out to explore women's primary health care needs, expectations and experiences of care as perceived by women users, non-users and professionals (Brooks, 1991; Brooks and Phillips, 1996; Phillips and Brooks, 1998). For this study 70 in-depth interviews were undertaken with women, and a random sample of 1251 women aged 16 to 65 years were surveyed by postal questionnaire on a wide range of issues relating to their use of and satisfaction with primary health care services. The study also incorporated an ethnographic exploration of women's experiences of community-based maternity care.

## Leading three or four lives: women's responsibilities and their health

Women's health cannot be understood independently of the social context within which it occurs (see for example Graham (1988) on smoking behaviour, Charles and Kerr (1988) on food). Women are much more likely than men to define health with reference to their social relationships, even if they are undertaking paid employment (Blaxter, 1990). Women are more likely than men to equate being healthy with being able to maintain or 'carry on' family relationships, such as having patience with children (Blaxter, 1990). Findings from the WPHC project indicated that women's definitions of health were mediated by their role in the maintenance and amelioration of the health of others. The majority of interviewees (52) stated unequivocally that the highest demands of caring fall on women. Of those who felt that women were the primary maintainers of family health, the overwhelming majority in the WPHC study felt this had a negative impact on women's health. For this group of women it was the context of women's lives, and specifically the responsibility for dependents and domestic labour, that was the greatest influence on the quality of women's health.

> Usually you put yourselves at the bottom of the heap and have to be nearly dead before you sort of drag yourself out of bed to make meals and things, and just take it as assumed that you'll carry on or else the place falls apart. You can't lie in bed. You just can't be ill.

> (woman, aged 54, two children, housewife)

The responsibility for maintaining the health of others means that women expend considerable emotional resources resolving the competing demands placed on their time and energy (Graham, 1984). Certainly, multiple roles can be a rewarding source of self-esteem, with potentially positive impacts on health (Annandale and Hunt, 2000).

However, studies of the health effects of domestic labour also indicate that the material demands of domestic labour are likely to be differently experienced and resolved according to women's access to economic resources (Popay, 1992) and the 'experienced quality' of those roles (Dennerstein, 1995).

Women interviewees recognised that competing demands had a cost in terms of their ability to maintain their own mental and physical health. Overall, the majority of women felt they were in a position in which they lacked the physical and emotional resources to enable them to prioritise their own health. Interviewees who were dependent on State benefits (22) overwhelmingly felt that their lack of material resources combined with their domestic responsibilities to ensure that it was particularly difficult to adopt a healthy lifestyle.

> I mean I've tried exercise and I can't do it without the kids climbing all over me. As for diet, diet is again very hard; there are pressures on you from other sources. They want their sweet things and my husband, if he ate health foods, he would disappear.

> (woman, aged 44, two children, factory worker)

Overall, women report higher levels of stress than men and have access to lower levels of social support to cope with stressful situations (Dengler et al. 1994; Doyal, 1998). In fact, for women stress may be a more significant health issue than reproductive health (Charles and Walters, 1994). Stress is also likely to be one part of the explanation as to why twice as many women as men receive psychiatric treatment in general practice (Payne, 1998).

> I see men getting very stressed with work, but again I see women who are very stressed with work, plus they've got their children to pick up and they've got two or three things to try and juggle round to do. Women do tend, from my experience, to have three or four lives to live at the same time really, and I think that's possibly why they end up very stressed. I mean, men do rather well out of getting married and having families.

> (woman, aged 29, no children, information officer)

*You spend a lot of time juggling your life: you know can I go to work,
when I get home I've got this to do. You never really get much chance to
be on your own and just be yourself.*

(woman, aged 34, two children, health care assistant)

Moreover, stress is likely to produce short-term coping strategies,
especially smoking and drinking (Charles and Walters, 1994).

*Well, men sort of, well mine, they go to work and they see to
themselves. A woman has gone to work, she's cleaned the house, she's
seen to the children. There's a lot more, it's a lot more complex for a
woman. There's a lot more involved. I mean a man decides to stop
smoking and it's just his will-power. A woman's got to battle with the
children getting aggravated.*

(woman, aged 49, three children, ex-secretary
now caring for a relative)

## Using the PHC services and reasoned decision-making

Women perceived there to be a connection between their multiple roles
and their usage of the PHC system, a connection that health care
professionals may not always understand. The comment from a GP at the
start of the chapter illustrates how high levels of consulting for
conditions that do not require physical treatment can lead to patients
being labelled 'heartsinks'. Moreover, the phenomenon of the 'heartsink'
patient also appears to be gender-related. Women, particularly those with
low levels of social support, have been perceived as both difficult by
health care providers (John *et al.* 1987) or as irrational and inappropriate
users of services (Roberts, 1992). In a context of lower social support and
multiple responsibilities, women's utilisation of the primary health care
service, even when consulting for apparently minor conditions, can be
seen to be based on appropriate and rational decision-making (Young,
1999).

*Men, when anything has happened they just take a few days in bed and
they get over it. Women tend to just carry on and therefore they'll go to*

*the doctor to give them something to enable them to carry on because they can't just go to bed for a few days.*

(woman, aged 40, two children, self-employed)

## Acknowledging the context of women's lives

**Question** *Is there anything more that GP practices could do?*

*I'm not sure how much they do actually. But I think it's something that should be done to help people under stress. I know they do it individually, but generally I don't know; general provision, I think that's something they could be doing.*

(woman, aged 60, two children, retired teacher)

Many women expressed the view that the service needed to both acknowledge, and be responsive to, the context of women's lives. A feature of the accounts was a need for the provision of broad preventive and health promotion services. This is a significant issue for primary care as, notable exceptions aside (Laughlin, 1998), many well-woman clinics have become almost exclusively focused around the cervical screening programme.

However, an understanding of the impact of the socio-economic context of women's lives was found to mark a starting point for a more sensitive and participative approach to the delivery of primary health care. For instance, a rejection by a midwife of individual pathology as the prime reason for non-adherence by many women to health promotion messages facilitated a more negotiated and potentially more effective approach to smoking in pregnancy.

*Like, many of the women just get by on cigarettes and being brave. So I don't tell them you must stop. I always say, 'Can you try and cut down?' I mean they do try; they know it is not good for the baby.*

(community midwife)

An understanding of material disadvantage also led another midwife to organise local 'natural childbirth' classes, while also acknowledging the complex and long-term nature of such an enterprise.

> **Question** *I have noticed that you never really mention NCT classes – is there any reason for that?*
>
> *I used to mention it all the time and the women would be keen, and then I would say, 'It is £20 or so and the nearest class is the other side of the city', and their faces would fall. So I run classes here, like the NCT ones with all the natural childbirth stuff. The ones who have come have been really keen and said it helped. But in an area like here it takes a long time for anything to really take off.*
>
> (community midwife)

## The ideal GP and pathways through information

Women were found to particularly value the provision of information and explanation about their health, although the form of communication women found to be useful was a far cry from traditional health education advice. When asked to identify the best aspects of their GP surgery, 'useful explanations from a GP' was valued by 40 per cent of the sample, and a GP who was 'easy to talk to' was the best aspect of their surgery for 54 per cent. 'Valuable communication with a GP' was clearly defined by women as a two-way process, one in which being able to contribute and being listened to was one of the most important aspects. Women also placed considerable value on professionals who supported them to gain pathways through medical knowledge. Access to medical notes is something that women particularly value and make active use of (Benato *et al.* 1998). Overall, the respondents' definition of what constituted a good general practice was determined by the extent of the professionals' willingness to share expertise and knowledge rather than just impart advice:

> *Well, somebody, who talks to you in a way that helps you ask the questions that you want to ask, or gives you as much information as possible, so that you know there isn't anything missed out. Sometimes*

*you feel that, unless you ask the right questions, they're not going to give you certain information. You have to ask it in a certain way.*

(woman aged 29, no children, clerical officer)

## Valuing shared decision-making

One obvious but often overlooked difficulty in involving patients in decision-making is that they are being asked to contribute when they may be feeling physically and psychologically vulnerable. The study identified several instances where women valued occasions when decision-making authority was assumed by a professional. However, most importantly, the sanction for this came from the women, and they actively chose to transfer decision-making to the professional. In the following example, the labouring woman's authority for the professional's judgement to predominate had been sought and given.

*Well, Helen [the midwife] said, 'I know you didn't want one, but I feel that if you don't you are likely to have a bad tear,' and I said, 'Fine'. I knew that she had made the right decision because that was what I needed.*

(woman aged 22–25, first child, shop worker)

In this context, the ability to influence or direct the management of a pregnancy or labour is bestowed on the professional by the woman, as someone who has the appropriate skills, rather than being assumed as a paternalistic, professional responsibility. This position appeared to be dependent upon two factors: first, that a good interpersonal relationship between provider and user had been established; and second, that the professional fully understood their views before transferring decision-making power.

When service users feel that decision-making has been achieved in partnership with health professionals, the responsibility for the risk and outcome of the decision may also become shared. In certain instances, where the outcome did not conform to the women's expectations, they were still able to retain a sense of control.

*Well, I was pushing for a long time, and Jean [the midwife] suggested that if she broke my membranes it might speed things up a bit. Well, I did feel tired so we thought that might be a good idea. But I still ended up pushing for another hour and the pain got really bad after that, because all the cushioning had gone. So I think we made the wrong decision on that one.*

(woman, aged 18–21, first child, bar worker)

## Challenges for women

In order for women to actively participate in health care decision-making they must be active agents in the decision-making process. Even so, there is comfort in the paternalistic father-figure of the doctor, despite the unequal power relationship. The image of the omnipotent caring professional is a very powerful one even when reality conflicts with that image. The following woman, when she first encountered a practice that encouraged active participation, felt daunted. Ultimately, she found the challenge to be something that enhanced feelings about her care:

*The attitudes of the GPs and practice nurses, the general consideration for people's feelings and thoughts, the shared decision-making; it is actually all a bit daunting at first, because it is so different to everywhere else. It is so unusual to everywhere else that you have to think, 'Oh, I have to make the decision now.' That is really daunting at first, but it is also very reassuring.*

(woman, aged 25, one child, unemployed)

## Conclusion: The future for women's voice in primary care

Through the use of accounts from women and practitioners, this chapter has highlighted that there is an important inter-relationship between the broader socio-economic context of women's lives, their health, and how they interact with the primary health care service.

Moreover, the narratives illustrate that an understanding of the rationality and context of women's health behaviours appears to facilitate shared decision-making and more effective care. Widespread acknowledgement of the importance of such an understanding is essential if primary care is to avoid reproducing gender-based inequalities in health. Initially, practitioners at the local level can do much by simply listening to women and developing an awareness of gender inequalities in their localities. The accounts from women indicate that many value the quality of interpersonal relationships with practitioners, and seek not only to be participants in the decision-making process, but to exercise control over it. In the past these areas have received relatively little attention in service planning and development (Doyal, 1998). Although the current policy represents a renewed opportunity in this direction, *The NHS Plan* explicitly acknowledges that 'many patients feel talked at, rather than listened to', and that there needs to be a shift towards shaping care around the concerns of patients (NHS Executive, 2000).

In order to address the concerns of women, gender divisions need to be understood as a variable in determining women's health. Plans for user involvement will need to ensure representation from women. Particular consideration needs to be given to how participation of women from minority ethnic communities can be achieved (Douglas, 1998). Ultimately, primary care's traditional capacity for innovative practice will be tested (Webb, 1984) if women are to be involved in exercising 'new powers and more influence over the way the NHS works' (NHS Executive, 2000).

## References

Annandale E, Hunt K. Gender inequalities and the social relations of gender. In: Annandale E, Hunt K, editors. *Gender inequalities in health*. Milton Keynes: Open University Press, 2000.

Benato R, Clarke A, Holt V, Lack V. Women and collective general practice: the Hoxton experience. In: Doyal L, editor. *Women and the Health Services*. Milton Keynes: Open University Press, 1998: 201–12.

Blaxter M. *Health and Lifestyles*. London: Routledge, 1990.

Brooks F. *Alternatives to the Medical Model of Childbirth: A Qualitative Study of User Centred Maternity Care*. PhD Thesis. Sheffield: University of Sheffield, 1991.

Brooks F, Phillips D. Do women want women health workers? Women's views of the primary health care service. Journal of Advanced Nursing 1996; 23: (6) 1207–11.

Charles N, Kerr M. *Women, Food and Families*. Manchester: Manchester University Press, 1988.

Charles N, Walters V. Women's health: women's voices. *Health and Social Care in the Community* 1994; 2 (6): 329–38.

Dengler R, Rushton L, Roberts H, Magowan R. Results from a lifestyle survey: Trent Health. *Health Education Research* 1994; 19 (3): 285–96.

Dennerstein L. Mental health, work and gender. *International Journal of Health Services* 1995; 25: 503–09.

Department of Health. *Changing Childbirth. Report of the Expert Maternity Group, Part 1*. London: HMSO, 1993.

Douglas J. Meeting the health needs of black and minority ethnic communities. In: Doyal L, editor. *Women and the Health Services*. Milton Keynes: Open University Press, 1998: 69–82.

Doyal L. Promoting Women's Health. In: Badura B, Kickbusch I, editors. *Health Promotion Research*. Geneva: WHO, 1991.

Doyal L. Conclusions the way forward. In: Doyal L, editor. *Women and the Health Services*. Milton Keynes: Open University Press, 1998: 238–50.

Graham H. *Women, Health and the Family*. Weston-Super-Mare: Harvester, 1984.

Graham H. Provider negotiators and mediators: women as the hidden carers. In: Lewin E, Oleson V, editors. *Women Health and Healing: Toward a new perspective*. London: Tavistock, 1985.

Graham H. Women and smoking in the United Kingdom: Implications for health promotion. *Health Promotion* 1988; 3 (4): 371–82.

Graham H. *Hardship and Health in Women's Lives*. Hemel Hempstead: Harvester, 1993.

John C, Schwenk T, Roi L, Cohen M. Medical care and demographic characteristics of 'difficult patients'. *The Journal of Family Practice* 1987; 24 (6): 607.

Kane P. *Women's Health: from womb to tomb*. London: St Martin's Press, 1991.

Laughlin S. From theory to practice: the Glasgow experience. In: Doyal L, editor. *Women and the Health Services*. Milton Keynes: Open University Press, 1998: 221–37.

Lyons C, Willott S. From suet pudding to superhero: Representations of men's health for women. *Health* 1999; 3 (3): 283–302.

NHS Executive. *The NHS Plan. A plan for investment. A plan for reform*. Cm 4818-I. London: The Stationery Office, 2000.

Payne S. 'Hit and miss': the success and failure of psychiatric services for women. In: Doyal L, editor. *Women and the Health Services*. Milton Keynes: Open University Press, 1998: 83–99.

Phillips D, Brooks F. Age differences in women's verdicts on the quality of primary health care services. *British Journal of General Practice* 1998; 48: 1151–54.

Popay J. My health is all right, but I'm just tired all the time: Women's experience of ill health. In: Roberts H, editor. *Women's Health Matters*. London: Routledge, 1992.

Roberts H. Professionals' and parents perceptions' of A&E use in a children's hospital. *The Sociological Review* 1992; 40 (1): 109–31.

Thomas P. Big boys don't cry? Mental health and the politics of gender. Editorial. *Journal of Mental Health* 1996; 5: 107–10.

Young I. Prioritising family health needs: a time-space analysis of women's health-related behaviours. *Social Science and Medicine* 1999; 48: 797–813.

Webb C. *Feminist practices in women's health care*. Chichester: Wiley, 1984.

Chapter 6

# Understanding user health care strategies: experiences of asthma therapy among South Asians and White cultural groups

Helen Lomax, Fiona Brooks and Martin Mitchell

## KEY POINTS

■ Patients engage in a range of self-management strategies. These include 'leaving off' prescribed medication and supplementing it with 'holistic' therapies.

■ Use of alternative therapies is common for all patients. However, the type of therapy used is contingent upon the ethnicity of the patient.

■ Where patients perceive that practitioners are disapproving of self-management strategies, they withhold information vital to the management of asthma and may cease to attend for asthma monitoring.

■ A therapeutic relationship based on collaboration and information exchange is preferred by patients and enables better management of asthma. Patients are able to bring important therapeutic information to the consultation and work with the practitioner to manage asthma. A key element of this approach is the recognition of the patient as an expert, ultimately responsible for his or her health.

## Introduction

*Well, the doctor is the most problematic thing at the moment. It seems like the doctors are overworked and there are a lot of people waiting to see them ... In those circumstances, the doctor does not have much time although you would like to talk to him, but you know he is not listening because his body language says, 'Look, this is what I'm prescribing for you.' He gives you a quick smile and then tells you to go away.*

(Indian respondent)

*He calls your name through a closed door. You go in and ... before you even sit down ... he writes your prescription and that's it.*

(White respondent)

Understanding the patient's perspective on his/her medication is central to an effective therapeutic relationship and management of illness (Marinker, 2000; Marinker, 1997; Mullen, 1997).

In relation to asthma, however, there has been little research into patients' self-management strategies, their impact on medication usage, and the degree to which discussion of these is a feature of the consultation. This chapter draws upon a recent qualitative study undertaken with South Asian and White asthmatics and a sample of health professionals working with these groups (Brooks, Mitchell and Lomax, 1999). Focusing on respondents' narratives concerning 'adherence' with prescribed medication, their use of alternative therapies and their relationships with providers, the analysis demonstrates the importance of incorporating users' perspectives in order to achieve a more effective therapeutic relationship and better management of asthma.

## The Asthma Research Project

In-depth interviews were conducted with 107 patients (Bangladeshi, n=17; Indian, n=33; Pakistani, n=30; and White, n=27) in non-medical settings in the language of patients' choice. The sample reflected the relative proportion of each ethnic group living in the south-east of England (Coleman and Salt, 1996). In addition, 20 health professionals (general practitioners, practice nurses, linkworkers, health visitors, school nurses and specialist asthma nurses) were interviewed to enable an exploration of practitioners' experience and awareness of patients' self-management strategies.

# Attitudes to prescribed medication

Patients' responses indicated a complex relationship with prescribed medication, a complexity that belies the traditional division of patients into compliers/non-compliers. While over half of respondents (55 per cent, n=59) reported that they took their medication as prescribed, it became apparent that 'non-compliance' was the dominant practice in our sample. Almost two-thirds (59 per cent, n=63) of patient interviewees reported that they sometimes reduced the dosage or 'left off' their prescribed medication, a figure that was comparable across ethnic groups:

> **Respondent:** *There are times when she is feeling better, when she isn't coughing a lot. Then I won't give her this [prescribed medication].*
> **Interviewer:** *When she is better then you don't give her any?*
> **Respondent:** *No, when she is better then I stop completely.*

> (Pakistani respondent talking about her 9-year-old child)

The prevalence of non-compliance was high (Marinker, 1997). However, it is worth highlighting that admissions of this style of medication usage were frequently obtained only after initial claims of taking medication as prescribed. This reluctance to admit non-standard medication usage indicated awareness that drug-taking might be perceived negatively by practitioners.

## Attitudes to prescribed medication: reasons for 'leaving off'

Both practitioners and patients were asked to explore reasons for stopping prescribed medication. Table 6.1 below illustrates the top three explanations given by professionals and patients.

**Table 6.1** Top three reasons for 'leaving off' prescribed medication

| Patients | Health professionals |
| --- | --- |
| Feeling well (48%) | Feeling well (70%) |
| Side effects (28%) | Difficulty using inhalers (65%) |
| Fear of dependency (14%) | Ignorance (60%) |

'Feeling well' was cited as an important reason for 'leaving off' both by practitioners (70 per cent) and by patients (48 per cent) across each of the ethnic groups sampled. However, the responses actually represent a divergence in understanding between the two groups. As the following quotations illustrate, while patients' responses indicate a calculated decision based on their lived experience of symptoms, practitioners tended to perceive them as deriving from ignorance:

> **Respondent:** Sometimes I can afford not to take my Becotide and my asthma is no problem.
> **Interviewer:** So it happens that you sometimes take less medicine and sometimes you take more? You reduce the dosage?
> **Respondent:** Yes. If I find that my asthma isn't a problem and I'm not using my Ventolin, then during the cooler months I can take lower doses of Becotide. It's not a problem.
>
> (White respondent)

> They feel better and they just think, 'I don't need it anymore.'
>
> (general practitioner)

The second most common reason given by patients for not taking medication as prescribed was concern about side effects (28 per cent of whole sample). Respondents reported anxiety about steroids and experienced a range of side effects affecting digestion, the skin and nervous system. Concern was strongest amongst the Indian respondents (58 per cent, n=19).

In contrast to patient accounts, the second and third most frequently cited reasons for 'leaving off' by health professionals were 'difficulty using inhalers' and 'ignorance'. This is illustrated by the following quotation from a general practitioner:

> I don't think they understand ... You understand ... You know they don't. Simply you've got to actually drum it into them [about] how important it is and what the medication involves. I don't think half of them understand it.

The view that patients are unable to use their inhalers properly and are ignorant of their condition is not supported by patients' narratives. Patients' accounts demonstrated complex knowledge about the onset of their condition, triggers and medication regimens. In addition, 'forgetting' to take medication was mentioned by only eight patients as an explanation for not taking their prescribed medication. More frequently, respondents provided more complex explanations concerning feeling well, fear of dependency and side effects.

Very few South Asian asthma patients perceived any particular stigma attached to asthma or asthma therapies within their communities. Similarly, when asked about the impact of religion, respondents were at pains to point out that it had little impact on their medication usage:

> I believe in God but I still take my medicine.

> (Bangladeshi respondent)

## Use of alternative therapies

Use of alternative therapies was widespread and associated with 'leaving off' prescribed medication. Of the 63 respondents who reported 'reducing down' or 'leaving off', the majority (84 per cent, n=53) were also using a complementary or 'holistic' approach to asthma self-management (e.g. home remedies, diet or exercise therapy).

**Table 6.2** Percentage of sample engaging in 'alternative' approaches

Food avoidance (47%)
Exercise (36%)
Food inclusion (31%)
Home remedies (31%)
Aromatherapy (10%)
Chinese medicine (7%)
Homoeopathy (7%)

Although the sample was constructed for a small-scale qualitative study, there was little difference in the numbers using alternative therapies across ethnic groups, but there were striking differences in the nature of therapies used. South Asians as a whole were almost twice as likely than Whites to emphasise dietary and herbal remedies. Avoiding and/or including certain foods as a means of controlling asthma was a common practice among South Asian groups compared to a minority of the White group.

While patients from all groups emphasised the need for a 'healthy' diet to manage their symptoms, the types of food and drink avoided tended to reflect the ethnic and cultural influences of each group. Avoiding 'cold' drinks and oily foods was common to all the South Asian groups. Food avoidance for the South Asian respondents did not simply follow an arbitrary pattern but was linked to traditional ideas of 'hot' and 'cold'. While cold foods, or 'perji', such as ice cream and yoghurt, are avoided because of links with respiratory problems, spices such as ginger, turmeric and saffron are taken in warm drinks as a means of clearing the lungs. The concept is particularly associated with the Hindu population, but there was some evidence that it had spread into other communities. Whites, by contrast, mentioned no food or drink more than once. The few factors that were mentioned tended to be much more closely linked with the concept of 'allergy'. While these different approaches may reflect different cultural traditions, all groups talked about a desire to manage their asthma more 'holistically'.

### Discussing holistic approaches with health professionals: fear of disapproval

Many patients commented that they would not discuss their use of alternative medication with their practitioner. For some patients this was based on previous negative experiences of talking to their practitioner about the use of alternative remedies:

> **Interviewer:** *And had you told your doctor about the fact that you were using herbal medicine?*
> **Respondent:** *No, no, no, he wouldn't like it.*
> **Interviewer:** *He wouldn't?*

*Respondent: No. Well, I'd discussed it before with my doctor and he didn't like the idea of using, you know, herbal medicines.*

(Indian respondent)

In a minority of cases, fear of disapproval resulted not only in the curtailing of any discussion about self-management strategies but also in patients no longer consulting for asthma:

*Interviewer: So when you visited the homoeopath … did you discuss this with your doctor?*
*Respondent: No, no. I never went back to the doctor after that. He had been so unhelpful.*

(White respondent)

While these are extreme examples, they demonstrate the importance of keeping avenues of communication open between practitioner and patient. It is this point that the final section of the chapter will address.

## The therapeutic relationship: from compliance to concordance

The interviews with the health professionals revealed a range of strategies for managing the therapeutic relationship with patients. These can be conceptualised as 'instructive', 'informative' and 'partnership'.

### Instructive: comply – or die

This approach, which was described by a total of eight professionals, reflects a view of the professional as expert, with the patient expected to submit to his or her expertise. Patients, in this view, are expected to 'follow doctor's orders'. The professionals' role is to keep them on track. The patient as a partner, with opinions and expertise of his or her own, is not recognised:

*The main thing … regarding asthma management … is to be severe on compliance … that's the only way to keep tight control … We can't leave anything for the patient to dictate.*

(general practitioner)

Patients are expected simply to comply with doctor's orders; those who fail to do this are perceived as 'undisciplined' and 'forgetful':

> *They forget, they are lazy, they don't take it and they keep coming for [treatment] and I say, 'We can't treat you.' We say that, 'Either [take the medication as prescribed] or find somebody else. I'm not going to be responsible for your death.'*
>
> (general practitioner)

This reflects a paternalistic view of medicine in which medical knowledge is prioritised over 'lay' experience, and the experience of illness is expressed in a technical, biomedical frame of reference to the exclusion of the social and biographical context of patients' lives (Fisher, 1991). However, as a means of managing asthma it is limited. Faced with such an approach, patients feel intimidated and are unable to bring important therapeutic information to the consultation. As the following example illustrates, patients evaluate the benefits of taking medication against 'leaving off', while being aware, at the same time, that doctors are acting upon a different set of values:

> **Interviewer:** *So are you able to discuss these concerns with your doctor?*
> **Respondent:** *Well, if I tell them I don't take it they get very angry. I did … in December and he told me I was being very silly. 'If you took it,' he said, 'you wouldn't be here.' Well, for my one or two attacks a year I would rather not take it.*
>
> (White respondent)

A Bangladeshi patient who experienced a clash between her own cultural beliefs and those of her GP demonstrated one cultural dimension to these difficulties:

> **Interviewer:** *Have you told the doctor that you don't take that much medicine?*
> **Respondent:** *No. The doctor, when the doctor gave it, it was quite bad. Then, when I took medicine, our kind of medicine, then I noticed a*

*lot of improvement ... it got better and I stopped going to the doctor ... I don't go for asthma anymore.*

(Bangladeshi respondent)

These examples are indicative of the influence of patients' own experiences, including cultural beliefs, on medication usage and the importance of openness in the consultation. Operating in a way that prohibits discussion, practitioners fail to glean important information about patients' self-management strategies. This has important implications for the ability of the practitioner to manage the patients' asthma effectively.

## Informative: justifying the biomedical

This was the most common strategy for trying to manage asthma, mentioned by 17 of the health professionals. Like the previous approach, it also has a narrow pharmacological focus. However, unlike the instructive approach, it is focused on 'advising', 'educating', 'persuading', 'recommending' and 'convincing' patients about the efficacy of their medications:

*I mean that's what we would do really ... try and convince people that there was a value in complying.*

(general practitioner)

*On the whole I would just try to persuade them. Or prove it to them, you know, by getting them to do a peak flow chart and to take their medication regularly for a month, or two months, to prove that it is improving things.*

(practice nurse)

As with the previous model, there is little room in this perspective for the patients' experiences when they diverge from the practitioners'. Rather, it is about convincing the patient of the efficacy of the biomedical model over his or her lived experience. As this quotation illustrates, patients were well aware of, and resistant to, this approach. A particular concern was the feeling that their GP simply did not listen to them, and this was particularly the case where medication was felt to be not working or inappropriate:

> *I told my doctor they didn't work and the doctor said, 'No, you are wrong.' I said, 'I'm the one with the asthma and I'm telling you they don't work properly', and he said, 'It's in your mind, it's psychological.'*

> (White respondent)

Traditional education approaches improve patients' knowledge but have little impact on medication usage and morbidity (Hilton *et al.* 1986; Jenkinson *et al.* 1988). Patients have their own ideas about medicine, based on their experience of living with it. Attempts to 'educate' them otherwise have little effect.

## Partnership: marrying experience and biomedicine

This approach, which was mentioned by 11 health professionals, also emphasised the need to demonstrate the efficacy of treatments. The key difference was the positive value practitioners attached to patients' experiences, as these contain important therapeutic information that helps the practitioner and patient frame decisions about asthma management:

> *Compliance is a term I don't like … because it does take away the control from the patient, and if I were the patient I would want to decide what medications I thought were making a difference to me … I'd rather talk about making a partnership with the patient about what they are going to do. For example, some people don't find 'X drug' acceptable, it upsets them … they don't like it and it tastes horrible and [they ask] do they really need it? In those circumstances I try and make a therapeutic alliance with them … At the end of the day, if they are not going to use it, I have got to use something else. I've got to be flexible around their view.*

> (general practitioner)

A key element of this approach is the willingness of the practitioner to respond to the patient's perspective, including altering medication. There was also a greater acceptance of alternative approaches, and the recognition that, sometimes, particular medications were not working. The emphasis in this perspective was on the relationship between the professional and patient. 'Accessibility', 'trust' and 'partnership' were seen as essential to good asthma management:

*I think you have to work in partnership with them in every way and there's more to it than just prescribing.*

(health visitor)

Through 'flexibility' and 'compromise' it was felt that patients would be more likely to discuss their approaches to the management of their asthma, a view that was supported by our interviews with patients. Great value was attached to occasions when health professionals had taken the time to listen to concerns and to explain treatments. In these instances, improved control of asthma was attributed by the respondent to the partnership approach of their practitioner:

*Yes, I can talk properly, frankly and with an open mind, and [the] doctor listens to me and advises me. There is no problem talking to my doctor. Yes, I do trust in my doctor and I am happy with his treatment. He knows what he is doing and my child is getting relief with his medicine and feels better.*

(Indian respondent)

This was also supported by the interviews with practitioners:

*Sometimes we find that actually what we suggested hasn't worked very well. Heresy! But that's often true. The patients often know better than we do. I've got one well-educated patient who recently was telling me that steroids didn't work for him, and so on and so forth. So, okay, we went into this big routine, we did a peak flow diary, we brought him back several times and actually he was damned right.*

(general practitioner)

## Conclusion

Interviews with patients revealed that both 'leaving off' prescribed medication and the use of holistic therapies were important self-management strategies for patients. Despite the prevalence of these practices, the degree to which patients could admit to them within the consultation varied enormously, and depended upon the attitude of the practitioner.

Interviews with practitioners revealed three different approaches to asthma management: 'instructive', 'informative' and 'partnership'. Within the first of these approaches there is little or no scope for the patients' experience or expertise. Rather, patients are expected merely to comply; behaviour other than strict compliance is considered deviant.

The informative model is similarly wedded to the view of the doctor as expert, although, in this approach, patients are 'encouraged' to comply with prescribed medication through demonstration of the medication's efficacy. There was much evidence, from our interviews with patients, that both approaches engender a fear of disapproval of self-management strategies, in that the patient is prevented from bringing his or her experiences of asthma management where it differs from the medical view.

The third approach to asthma management, by contrast, recognises that patients engage in a range of self-management strategies. Rather than seeing these as an impediment to asthma management, the 'partnership' model enables patients to voice their beliefs and experiences. There was much evidence that this is preferred by patients and that practitioners are then in a better position to manage asthma. Ultimately, this approach is successful because it recognises the patient as an expert in his or her health care decisions, and rejects the concept of compliance in favour of a concordant alliance in which the patient has final jurisdiction.

## References

Brooks F, Mitchell M, Lomax H. *Managing Asthma: Attitudes to Asthma and Asthma Therapy Among South Asian Cultural Groups.* Research report No. 503. Luton: University of Luton, Institute for Health Services Research, 1999.

Coleman I, Salt J. *Ethnicity in the 1991 census. Demographic characteristics of the ethnic minority populations.* London: OPCS/HMSO, Vol. 1, 1996.

Donovan J, Blake D. Patient non-compliance: Deviance or reasoned decision making? *Social Science and Medicine* 1992; 34 (5): 507–13.

Fisher S. A Discourse of the Social: Medical Talk/Power Talk/Oppositional Talk? *Discourse and Society* 1991; 2 (2): 157–82.

Hilton S, Sibbald-Anderson H, Freeling P. Decision Making in Acute Asthma. *Journal of the Royal Society of Medicine* 1986; 75: 625–30.

Jenkinson D, Davison J, Jones S, Hawtin P. Comparison of the Effects of a Self-Management Booklet and Audio-Cassette for Patients with Asthma. *BMJ* 1988; 277: 267–70.

Marinker M. *What Do We Mean By Concordance?* Concordance Co-ordinating Group, Royal Pharmaceutical Society of Great Britain, 2000. Concordance web site: www.concordance.org

Marinker M. Writing Prescriptions Is Easy. Personal Paper. *BMJ* 1997; 314: 787.

Mullen P. Compliance Becomes Concordance: Making a Change in Terminology to Produce a Change in Behaviour. *BMJ* 1997; 314: 691.

Royal Pharmaceutical Society of Great Britain. *From Compliance to Concordance: towards shared goals in medicine taking.* London: RPSGP, 1997.

Chapter 7

# Involving users with mental health problems

Angela Greatley

### KEY POINTS

■ Primary care is likely to be most effective when individuals play a part in planning their own care.

■ Primary Health Care Teams should involve users in staff training to improve the quality of mental health provision.

■ Users can identify the gaps. Their involvement can assist primary and specialist health and social care professionals produce better integrated systems of mental health care.

## Introduction

People with mental health problems are regular and significant users of primary care. They present a wide range of mental health problems to GPs and other members of Primary Health Care Teams (PHCTs). Their problems may be severe and complex or time-limited and relatively uncomplicated to treat. Any mental health difficulty can cause considerable distress to an individual or carer and can create demanding work for health professionals. Effective user involvement can make a real difference to this picture.

It is particularly important that users are involved in planning mental health services, whether these are primary, secondary or tertiary. When people become involved in shaping care they gain confidence in the treatments offered and this can increase the benefit they gain. In the treatment of mental health problems, participation can have positive therapeutic outcomes and be the key to emotional well-being (Hickey and Kipping, 1998). For some people it can even make the difference between engaging with mental health services or avoiding those services until a crisis occurs or, in very rare cases, tragedy strikes.

Individuals with mental health problems should play a part in planning their own care. They need to know what the options are and need to agree with practitioners as to the best way forward. This is now much more widely recognised in both primary care and in specialist services. For this chapter the term 'specialist services' will be used to encompass both secondary and tertiary mental health care.

Users of specialist services must be given the opportunity to take part in their own care planning through the Care Programme Approach (CPA) and local authority care management. These processes require statutory agencies to afford individuals the opportunity to take part in devising care plans. Whilst no such requirements are laid at the door of primary care, it is clearly good practice to involve users in determining their treatment and care.

> We are all the primary experts on our own mental health and about what works for us. (The Mental Health Foundation, 2000)

When individual service users combine, they can comment on quality, inform service development and bring about more responsive services. Users will often have experience of how the whole mental health system functions and of the patient's journey through health and social care. They are often best placed to say whether the system functions effectively and where the gaps are.

To date, experience of involving users in primary care mental health has been limited, but there are lessons to be learned and pointers to success at practice and team level and, more recently, at Primary Care Group (PCG) and Primary Care Trust (PCT) level. Some of these are raised in this chapter.

## What are the policies and how do they affect us?

Government has made mental health a major priority for improvement in health and social care. In its vision for a new kind of service, 'primary care plays a central role' (Department of Health, 1998). The National Service Framework for Mental Health (NSF) seeks to address problems with the quality of mental health services and variation in types of provision across the country in primary and specialist care.

The NSF sets standards in five areas of mental health service and includes primary care. For primary care, the standards concern identification and assessment of individual need, and emphasise the need to offer treatments of known effectiveness. There is also a standard requiring the provision of an appropriate response 'round the clock' (Department of Health, 1999). The emphasis is on responsive, timely and effective services that are sensitive to varying cultural needs. Commissioners and providers must ensure that specific arrangements are in place for user and carer involvement. One of the performance measures for monitoring success in implementing primary care mental health standards is the 'experience of service users and carers, including those from black and minority ethnic communities' (Department of Health, 1999).

For many years mental health policy has developed alongside primary care policy, but this has not happened in a co-ordinated fashion. A gap persists, with a sharp divide between primary and specialist care: between most people with mental health problems and 'the severely mentally ill'. But the position is changing. It is now likely that PCTs will be commissioners of specialist mental health services, and some may become providers, managing community mental health teams. This position will vary according to a number of factors. For example, PCTs in rural areas may take on greater responsibility for the provision of specialist community-based mental health care in order to ease acknowledged problems of patient access. If PCTs are to provide specialist care, the NSF is clear that they must meet a number of specific criteria. One is that they 'command the broad support of local users' (Department of Health, 1999). PCTs will need to develop strategies to seek the views and involvement of people with mental health problems in developing services, monitoring quality and influencing decisions about service configuration.

## Can primary mental health care make a difference?

It is estimated that mental health problems play some part in one-fifth to one-quarter of daily consultations in the surgery (Thornicroft and Strathdee, 1996; Tyrer et al. 1993). Around 90 per cent of the people who go to their GP and have a mental health problem identified will have their needs met in primary care. No more than 10 per cent will be referred to specialist mental health services. Improvements in the quality and range of the mental health provision delivered in primary care can make a real difference to the lives of up to one-quarter of those who come to the surgery.

However, we cannot discount the primary health care needs of people who are referred for specialist care, since a large number of them will continue to use primary care services as well. Increasingly, some elements of specialist mental health care are delivered in the community. In future this may involve more specialist staff, for example community mental health nurses working within primary care practice premises. It may also mean that primary care staff offer more shared care packages with specialist teams. Many people with mental health problems also suffer physical illness. The physical health needs of those with mental illnesses are often overlooked and should be given higher priority.

## Where are the users?

At this stage we need to enter a note of caution. The last 20 years have seen the rise of a movement to get the views of mental health service users heard nationally and locally. There is a growing body of literature setting out user perspectives. However, most of the published material concerns user views of specialist services. Where we have views on primary care, these are often obtained from those who also use specialist mental health services. More research is undoubtedly required if we are to gain the views of those whose needs are met entirely within primary care mental health services (Gell, 1996).

Primary care practitioners and teams wanting to explore user views will find it helpful to discuss the availability of existing information with colleagues in health authorities, trusts, local authorities and PCGs. There may be existing material on user views of local primary care. It is important to take this into account.

## What users want from primary care

Mental health users' views were sought as part of a project funded by the Department of Health 'Building Partnerships for Success' programme (Greatley and Peck, 1999). Working with community mental health teams and GP practices in three areas of London, contact was also made with established user groups. Their key concerns about primary care can be summarised as follows:

- People want clear basic information about mental health problems.
- Communication between staff is sometimes poor and users fear that their own care will suffer as a result.
- Everyone should be treated decently when they go the local surgery, but people with mental health problems may not be.
- Most users would be happy to see a range of primary care professionals delivering their treatment.
- Some users would value the development of a range of alternative treatments and complementary services in primary care locations.

## Better information

*You see everything about having a baby and getting immunised, but it is like mental health stuff is shameful.*

Users want to see more written information about mental health conditions for them and for their carers. Often there is no written material in surgeries and some users spoke about the prohibitive costs of buying leaflets for themselves. There is a pressing need to deliver information in a different way for people who do not speak English as their first language or who find written material difficult to handle.

## Improving communication

*Sometimes it feels like I am the only channel of communication between my psychiatrist and the GP, and I worry about whether even the information on my medication is right.*

Users want to know that staff share regular channels of communication. This can mean anything from using quicker ways of transmitting key details between primary and secondary care, for instance on medication prescribed by the psychiatrist, through to changing the system for the CPA so that it becomes less bureaucratic for users – and for primary care professionals.

## A decent reception

*People are sympathetic if they see you've got a disability, but if its mental health it's invisible ... they see me as a nuisance.*

Users sometimes feel stigmatised by their treatment in the surgery. They think that they are ignored or, worse, seen as less desirable both by other patients and by reception staff. They feel that primary care staff are not properly trained to understand basic issues about mental illness. Some users spoke of the effects of being labelled as mentally ill and of their problems not being taken seriously by surgery staff.

*If you've got a psychiatric label no-one wants to hear about physical problems ... You're not taken seriously.*

People from ethnic minorities need advocacy and interpreting services in order to use primary care services and participate in decisions about their own treatment.

## Consultation and support

*It's still name/address/prescription.*

Mental health problems can feel very pressing to users and it seems that primary care is not always geared up to responding quickly or giving sufficient time. Users know that GPs and other staff are very busy and do not want to become nuisances. However, they want reassurance and advice, for instance about issues such as medication and side effects. They may be worried about taking the time of the doctor but also feel very rushed during consultations. They fear 'being struck off'.

Users are often happy to see different members of the PHCT and may be quite content to receive advice and information from nursing and other staff.

## New ways of working

*You don't always want to go through the door marked 'mental illness'.*

Many users value primary care and its potential for improving their treatment and care. Primary care is close to home: it involves fewer long – and expensive – journeys. Primary care is also used by everyone in the community and can really help to engage those who fear being labelled as mentally ill. This can be particularly important for some people from black and minority ethnic communities, for example young mothers from South Asian communities. Users would like to have more treatments delivered in primary care locations, for instance out-patient psychiatric clinics and psychological therapies.

Some people would like to be able to access other services, for instance welfare advice, advocacy and self-help groups. Some would welcome alternative approaches too, for instance aromatherapy or massage. Complementary therapies may be of particular importance for people from ethnic minority communities.

## Criticism and praise

These views echo research findings about user views of general practitioners, where further concerns are raised about labelling, stigma, and the difficulty of getting serious consideration for physical problems (Pilgrim and Rogers, 1993). They speak of not being listened to and of finding it difficult to establish trusting relationships with primary care (Bailey, 1997), and they worry that primary care staff rarely reviewed care plans and prescriptions in consultation with specialist practitioners (Gell, 1996).

However, users in most studies also recognise the value of good primary care (Pilgrim and Rogers, 1993). GPs are often seen in 'a more favoured light' than psychiatrists and 'seem to prefer treatment in primary rather than secondary care settings'.

## Must changes to mental health care always be put on the 'too difficult' pile?

Whilst primary care professionals have legitimate concerns about working with specialist teams, the specialist health services and social care agencies often report difficulties in working with primary care. There are concerns about communication, about a lack of understanding of different professional and agency practices, about the quality of primary care, and about pressure to deliver services in practice premises.

These problems have proved remarkably persistent. Involving users and gaining their views could be one of the keys to unlocking the doors marked 'too difficult' in the system of mental health care.

## Help to tackle change

There is a growing body of literature on how primary care can work with specialist mental health services and with social care to address long-standing difficulties (some are referred to later in this section). If adopted, there are many changes that will bring about direct benefits for users. However, if the users themselves become involved, even greater improvement may be achieved.

In some cases officers and members of PCG and PCT boards will have little direct experience of mental health needs or services. They may need to set up mechanisms by which they can become more familiar with the issues and set mental health in its broader context. This can be achieved by arranging joint 'awareness' sessions involving health and local authorities, trusts and key user representatives.

There are useful texts for PCGs and PCTs, providing systematic guidance on Health Improvement Programmes, commissioning, partnership working, developing primary mental health care, and integrating primary and community care (Cohen and Paton, 1999). Lessons can also be learned on improving collaboration between primary care and social services from work concerning care for older people (Rummery and Glendinning, 2000).

Individual practices and groups of practices in an area may already be working together to address the needs of people with long-term mental health problems. Finding out about existing initiatives and joining in with colleagues may be a way forward for some. This kind of initiative can improve team working, develop inter-professional and inter-agency training, and tackle difficulties in communication within and between services providers. Some practices will work to develop shared care arrangements, including improving the delivery of CPA and care management, and developing protocols and guidelines. Others may want to update information on medication and develop guidance on self-medication. Whatever the initiative, it can be shared using mechanisms developed by PCGs and PCTs. Practical guidance on many of these issues can be found in *Developing Primary Care for Patients with Long-term Mental Illness* (Byng and Single, 1999).

## How can we work with users?

Involving people with mental health problems in planning their own care should help them to get the right kind of service. Users are often well placed to know how the system can be improved. Mental health care is a large and complex system that relies on the effective working of each component part, for example good primary care and good social care. But the development of the whole system also requires integration of the component parts. Users often know where the problems are and can suggest how to fix them. It is likely that new ways can be found to resolve long-standing difficulties between primary care, specialist health care and social care by starting from a user perspective.

### Where are we aiming to be?

There are many ways of demonstrating the 'changing interfaces between the users of mental health services, their carers and the staff' (The NHS Advisory Service, 1997). The following is one illustration of how this might develop:

- No user involvement – judgements are professionally/managerially based.
- Information and advice – are offered about entitlements and how to use services.
- Consultation – users consulted, but decisions remain with professionals/managers.

- Involvement – users asked views and given opportunities to influence decisions.
- Joint working – users given information and support to participate in decision-making.
- Users empowered – taking control of planning and managing services.

Whilst effective user empowerment – with users exercising power in the decision-making process and over the delivery of care – is a long way from where most services are, or aspire to be, movement in that direction is desirable.

## Limitations

There are, however, many differences between users and one approach will not suit all.

- Some fear prejudice and may not join patient groups, but will offer views through written surveys or confidential discussion.
- Some find it difficult to speak with professionals, but will talk with other users.
- Some will dominate meetings to the detriment of other users and this may require careful facilitation.
- Some are worried that their care will suffer if they seem critical of their GP or practice staff, but will talk in broadly based groups where comments are more generally applicable.

Users do want to be involved but they are sensitive to how much time is taken up in consultation and joint planning. (One woman at a recent conference was worried that her GP was always 'going to these groups' and might not have time to see her.) Users and professionals will need to strike a balance.

## Prepare carefully and take practical steps

Start simply; a first step might be to review the quality and range of written material in practices. A practice or group of practices might commission translations of material into appropriate community languages. These issues are important because good clear information reduces patient anxiety, gives a sense of control, and enables users and carers to discuss problems. An established local user group can help practices in this task.

Use health open days, health fairs and similar events to acquire community views about local mental health problems. The problems may not be labelled 'mental health', but much useful information can be obtained in this way. This will help PCG/Ts to build up a profile of mental health needs and services, adding to what health, local authorities and trusts can provide.

Identify the user groups that operate locally. Social services contacts, specialist services and health authorities are well placed to help in this. Once contact has been established, find out what work has already been done about primary care. Building upon what is known will save time and will help reassure users that PCG/Ts do not mean 'starting all over again'.

Involve users in training practice staff. Individuals will need support to participate in this kind of work, and such support may be offered by a patient or user group.

PCGs and PCTs start in very different places regarding mental health. Some need to make initial contact with users; others can draw on a wealth of local experience. The PCG lay member may or may not be experienced in mental health issues, but, whatever his/her background, should not be left to carry the burden alone (see Chapter 3). A reference group or user panel may be needed to offer advice on a regular basis.

There have long been problems in getting the voice of the primary care mental health user heard. There are also long-standing difficulties in achieving collaboration between health and social care. User involvement can be the key to improving primary care and to improving collaboration.

## References

Bailey D. What is the way forward for a user-led approach to the delivery of mental health services in primary care? *Journal of Mental Health* 1997; 6 (1): 101–05.

Byng R, Single H. *Developing Primary Care for Patients with Long-term Mental Illness*. London: King's Fund, 1999.

Cohen A, Paton J. *A Workbook for Primary Care Groups*. London: The Sainsbury Centre for Mental Health/Royal College of General Practitioners, 1999.

Department of Health. *Modernising Mental Health*. London: 1998.

Department of Health. *National Service Framework for Mental Health*. London: 1999.

Gell C. User involvement in primary care. *The Mental Health Review* 1996; 1: 3.

Greatley A, Peck E. *Mental Health Priorities for Primary Care*. London: King's Fund, 1999.

Hickey G, Kipping C. Exploring the concept of user involvement in mental health through a participation continuum. *Journal of Clinical Nursing* 1998; 7: 83–88.

Pilgrim D, Rogers A. Mental health service users' views of medical practitioners. *Journal of Interprofessional Care* 1993; 7 (2).

Rummery K, Glendinning C. *Primary Care and Social Services: Developing New Partnerships for Older People*. The National Primary Care Research and Development Centre Series. Abingdon: Radcliffe Medical Press, 2000.

The Mental Health Foundation. *Strategies for Living*. London: 2000.

The NHS Health Advisory Service. *Voices in Partnership*. Williams E, Emerson G, Muth Z, editors. London. The Stationery Office, 1997.

Thornicroft G, Strathdee G. *Commissioning Mental Health Services*. London: HMSO, 1996.

Tyrer P, Higgs R, Strathdee G. *Mental Health and Primary Care*. London: Gaskell/The Mental Health Foundation, 1993.

Chapter 8

# Carers' contribution in primary care

Penny Banks

### KEY POINTS

■ Government policy gives primary health care a key role in identifying and supporting carers, who are partners in providing care and who have needs in their own right.

■ Given their unique role, with expertise in caring and experience of using services, carers make a vital contribution towards planning, evaluating and developing primary health care services.

■ Primary health care can draw upon considerable experience of successfully involving carers in planning and developing services. There is evidence that where carers' issues are being embedded into the way organisations operate, change is taking place.

■ Although there are a number of examples where prompts and checks are being built into primary care systems, there is still some way to go to ensure mainstream practice consistently addresses the needs of carers and recognises their contribution.

## Introduction

The importance of care provided by family, partners and friends has been increasingly recognised over the last decade. For every 1000 patients in a practice population, it is estimated there will be 120 carers supporting relatives or friends because of illness, disability or frailty. It is likely that just over 40 per cent of the carers will be men. A large proportion of the carers will be aged between 45 and 64, but there will also be children supporting family members. The personal and emotional care that unpaid carers provide treatment and 24-hour supervision is valued at nearly £34 billion per annum (Nuttall *et al.* 1994), and could never be replaced by health and social care services.

This major contribution has been acknowledged in recent government policy, which aims to enable 'those who choose to care, and where care is wanted by another person, to do so without detriment to carers' inclusion in society and to their health'. The first national strategy for carers, *Caring about Carers* (1999), directs all organisations to focus not just on the client, patient or user, but also to include carers. Primary health care is given a key role in identifying carers and providing them with information, sign-posting to support services, and helping carers to maintain their own health. The strategy also stresses that carers are key partners in providing care and have an important contribution to service planning and development.

Thus, carers are significant to primary health care, first, as they are partners with experience of using services and with expertise in caring, and second, because they are an investment. Not only is it cost-effective to support carers who provide long-term care and can prevent patients unnecessarily returning to hospital (Castleton, 1998), but practices that have supported carers report a drop in their anti-depressant drugs bill and decreased consultation rates (Warner, 1999). Third, carers are 'patients' too, and primary care has responsibilities towards carers whose own health may be at risk because of their caring responsibilities. Indeed, many carers are elderly, or approaching old age, and have their own health problems. A recent national survey (Henwood, 1998) found more than half of all carer respondents were looking after other people while experiencing substantial physical or psychological ill health of their own. Back and upper limb problems, stress and depression are frequently reported.

Carers from all communities see primary care as a crucial point of contact. They are likely to turn to their GP or community nurse as a first port of call to seek advice, information or help. Henwood shows that 72 per cent of carers rated their GP as the most powerful member of NHS staff, followed by district and community nurses (Henwood, 1998).

This chapter will give examples of carer involvement in primary health care, both in planning and service development, and in front-line practice as individuals with needs of their own. The examples draw extensively upon the recent national development programme 'Carers Impact', which was led by the King's Fund (1996–99). 19 sites across the country took part in the programme, including members of primary care services in each location. Over 500 carers were involved in local work to improve services (Banks and Cheeseman, 1999).

## Involving carers in planning and developing services

'Carers Impact' demonstrated the benefits of involving carers in improving local services. Practitioners and managers from primary care, acute trusts, health and local authorities, and voluntary organisations worked with carers to improve local services. Rather than 'opening the floodgates', as feared by some staff, clear benefits were identified by all the agencies working alongside carers. These included:

- Better understanding by all the professionals of the real needs of carers – not always resource intensive.
- Freeing-up of agency boundaries and encouraging a 'whole systems' approach that assisted planning.
- Sharing a wide range of expertise, experiences and perspectives, which encouraged more lateral and imaginative thinking.
- Immediate feedback from carers' experiences of policies, services and practices to assist in standard setting and monitoring.

### Case example 1 – 'Taking stock and taking action' workshops

The 'Carers Impact' programme successfully involved carers in reviewing local services by holding a special workshop with carers, practitioners and managers from primary and acute health care, local authority and voluntary organisations. The workshops were carefully planned to ensure all key stakeholders participated. Carers were fully prepared beforehand, where necessary with special pre-briefing meetings. The workshops were devised to:

- **Develop shared ownership** through exercises designed to map out local work, thereby ensuring both personal and organisational experiences could be shared.

- **Form a common value set** through debating the underlying principles and collectively drawing together a picture of the 'ideal future'.

- **Encourage all participants to take responsibility beyond the workshops** through agreeing priorities and developing action plans. Review workshops were held a year later, again with carers involved, to see what progress had been made and to update plans.

- **Streamline cross-cutting planning** and provide an approach that made sense to carers who were not caught up in agencies' divisions of responsibilities.

## Case example 2 – Linking into carer networks

Some authorities have supported the development of carer networks, which can provide invaluable two-way communication between services and carers, as well as between carers.

In one authority, a Carers' Council, elected by carers, communicates with over ten different neighbourhood carer support groups, and has a direct voice into joint strategic work between health, social and community services. Carers from the local Asian community are encouraged to take part by the local authority, who employ bilingual workers to go out into the community and literally 'knock on doors'.

A carer nominated by the Carers' Council takes part on one of the sub-groups of the Primary Care Group (PCG) and is supported by the carer network, so perspectives from a wide range of caring situations and communities can be fed into the discussions. This avoids the pitfalls of token representation by one or two carers at planning meetings. The PCG has thus been able to key into established carer networks. The involvement of carers from the Carers' Council has also motivated individual general practices to review their approach to carers.

## Case example 3 – Going out to carers

Involving carers in meetings is only one way of engaging with carers to improve services. Some managers of primary care services ensure they go out regularly to speak to carers in their own homes as well as visit carers who meet together in support groups. For example, as part of their supervisory responsibilities, nursing managers in one community trust undertake periodic visits to carers. This provides important opportunities for managers to hear directly about their experiences of services.

Some general practices and health centres run their own carer groups, either supported by primary care staff or by special carer support link-workers. These groups not only provide peer support to carers but can also provide a forum to feedback comments and concerns about services.

## Good practice checklist

In summary, the experiences of the sites taking part in the 'Carers Impact' programme highlighted the following well-rehearsed issues that need to be addressed to ensure an effective engagement with carers. There needs to be:

**(a) Clarity and shared expectations between all the partners as to**

- the nature of the engagement and what it is trying to achieve
- timescale, ensuring adequate time to involve carers properly
- roles and responsibilities of all the partners
- who will make decisions and what the outcome will be.

**(b) Recognition that no one individual can represent all the carers, instead**

- two-way communication needs to be developed with wider carer and community networks
- an on-going dialogue needs to be created outside of clinical interventions between carers and managers, practitioners and staff. A range of approaches can be taken, for example using newsletters, feedback phonelines, visiting community and carer groups, holding carer panels, speaking to carers in their own homes.

**(c) Support to take part, for example**

- sensitive facilitation so that carers have an equal voice and everyone is kept fully informed throughout the process
- practical support, such as expenses and substitute care
- training or briefings for carers
- interpreters or support to carers with any special needs.

**(d) Regular reviews of progress and feedback, in order to**

- identify any changes made as a result of carer involvement
- involve any new members.

## Involving carers as individuals and partners

Carers occupy an ambiguous position in relation to services, in that 'they lie on the margins of the social care system; in one sense within its remit, part of its concerns and responses; in another, beyond its remit, part of the taken-for-granted reality against which welfare services operate'. (Twigg *et al.* 1994) There are tensions between the Government's commitment to support carers and State expectations of family responsibilities (Olsen, 1997). Indeed, there is no clear consensus as to how much care family members should undertake, whether they should be given any real choice, at what point they can expect some help, and what minimum level of support should be provided.

These ambiguities and other pressures on front-line staff working within tight budget constraints have resulted in very different responses to the needs of carers (Banks, 1999). Carers may be seen simply as a resource to help hard-pressed staff carry out their responsibilities, rather than as individuals with needs of their own. Whilst central policy has made it clear that 'carers have a right to expect that the NHS and social services should help them to maintain their health' (Department of Health, 1999), and underlines the important role for primary care in identifying, informing and training carers, there is still room for very different individual interpretation, particularly in the absence of explicit local guidelines. Many health professionals do not know about the Carers (Recognition and Services) Act 1995, nor do they advise carers that they may be entitled to an assessment of their own needs.

Confidentiality is frequently cited as a major obstacle for doctors and other health professionals in their relationship with carers. To address this, government policy promotes a proactive approach to offering help and information by general practitioners and clinicians, so that they 'always explicitly seek the patient's consent for information to be passed to their carer'. (Department of Health, 1999) In the majority of cases where the patient has a carer, the patient is happy for their carer to know as much as *they* do. Where patients refuse to consent to any information being given to their carer, central policy recommends that decisions about providing information in the interests of individual or public safety would have to be taken on the basis of each individual case.

Conflicts between the patient and carer can be problematic for front-line staff who feel torn between loyalties to both 'sides'. They are particularly evident in the field of mental health and learning difficulties. Sensitive negotiation to find a solution can take time and in some situations may need an independent advocate to free-up discussions.

Despite the policy contradictions and challenges to introduce patient-centred and carer-friendly practice, there is some evidence that carers are beginning to move up, or at least onto, the agenda of primary care. A recent analysis undertaken by the King's Fund of all local authority plans to use the Carers Special Grant found one-third of authorities made reference to work on carers' issues with PCGs (Banks and Roberts, 2000).

Whilst mixed results have been reported by carer support workers who have a special remit to work with primary care (Clark, 1997), there is some evidence that, where carers issues are being embedded into the way organisations operate, change is taking place and carers' contributions are being properly recognised (Banks and Cheeseman, 1999). This goes beyond carer awareness training for practitioners and staff, and is where prompts and checks are built into the system to ensure carers are part of mainstream practice.

## Examples of primary care systems recognising carers' contributions

- Carers issues are clearly addressed within Health Improvement Programmes and Primary Care Investment Plans.
- All staff, including receptionists, receive carer awareness training at induction, and periodic staff questionnaires or communications

review staff knowledge of carer developments, provide staff with information, and seek staff views on practice and service developments relating to carers.

- Some primary care teams have nominated a 'carer champion' who undertakes to keep the team updated on carer issues and service information, and to keep carers high on the agenda. In some areas this champion is supported by carer organisations or carer support projects.
- Some general practices and primary care teams now have recording systems in place to identify carers and alert all staff to monitor the carer's health, and proactively provide information and signpost carers to support services (to meet national priorities guidance).
- Protocols have been established to refer carers to social services for carer assessments and to other agencies such as housing, carer support organisations and benefits advice.
- Supervisory responsibilities include checks to ensure staff have involved carers and given them information.
- New patient health checks and registration, and over-75s health checks are used as key points to identify and contact carers.
- All information provided by primary care teams includes references to carers; for example, public noticeboards, practice leaflets, appointment cards and messages with repeat prescriptions.
- Special appointments are reserved for carers at the beginning of surgeries to ensure they can attend.

## Conclusion

There are dangers that the new emphasis on carers becomes little more than an added paragraph on policy documents or that carers are simply bracketed with users. Although there is a substantial shared agenda between patients and carers, the unique position of carers calls for a clear strategy for their involvement so that their distinct needs are properly addressed and their special contribution recognised. Carers need opportunities to have their say separately from the people they support.

Primary care professionals can draw on considerable experience of involving carers and can usefully link into local networks already in place. The challenge remains to build on and improve local involvement, to engage with those who do not readily identify with the term 'carer', and to reach out to these people who may be some of the most socially excluded.

## References

Banks P. *Carer Support: Time for a change of direction?* London: King's Fund, 1999.

Banks P, Cheeseman C. *Taking Action to Support Carers: A Carers Impact guide for commissioners and managers.* London: King's Fund, 1999.

Banks P, Roberts E. *A Break for Carers? An analysis of local authority plans to use the Carers Special Grant.* London: King's Fund, 2000.

Castleton B. *Developing a Whole System Approach to the Analysis and Improvement of Health and Social Care Services for Older People and their Carers: A pilot study in West Byfleet, Surrey.* (unpublished MS), 2000.

Clark W. *Nobody Asked Me: A review of a GP/Carers Project.* London: London Borough of Sutton, 1997.

Department of Health. *Caring about Carers: A National Strategy for Carers.* London: The Stationery Office, 1999.

Henwood M. *Ignored and Invisible? Carers' experience of the NHS.* London: Carers National Association, 1998.

Olsen R. Carers and the missing link: Changing professional attitudes. *Health and Social Care in the Community* 1997; 5 (2): 116–23.

Nuttall S R *et al.* Financing Long-Term Care in Great Britain. *Journal of the Institute of Actuaries* 1994; 121, Part 1: 1–68.

Twigg J, Atkin K. *Carers Perceived: policy and practice in informal care.* Milton Keynes: Open University Press, 1994.

Warner L. *Seven and a half minutes is not enough.* London: The Princess Royal Trust for Carers, 1999.

Chapter 9

# Developing services with older people

Margaret Edwards

**KEY POINTS**

■ In the past, older people have often been excluded from consultations on service development. They are, however, interested and able to participate in local discussions about services.

■ PCGs and PCTs should work jointly with other local statutory and voluntary organisations when involving older people, both to avoid duplication and to reinforce partnership.

■ Forward planning can ensure that getting involved is made easy for older people.

■ Older people can contribute views on the whole system of local services and will be especially interested in community services.

## Introduction

Central to the Government's modernisation agenda for public services is an emphasis on involving the public in contributing to plans for change, particularly at a local level. On average, as people age they tend to make greater use of health and social care services. Data produced by the Audit Commission (1997) shows that those aged over 65 years constitute 14 per cent of the population and account for 47 per cent of Department of Health expenditure. The activities of PCGs are especially relevant to older people because they have the potential to identify local health needs and allocate funding accordingly.

Government policy is influenced by evidence that older people, in particular, tend to be excluded from participation in decision-making about services designed for them, as well as from mainstream social activities. In a Department of Social Security publication (1998), Tony Blair states:

*to meet its goals, the Government needs older people to be fully involved*
*in deciding priorities and helping shape the policies to meet them.*

This paper draws on an analysis of consultation events that were organised by four different PCGs in co-operation with their partner agencies in health, local government and the voluntary sector during the early part of 2000. The events related to services provided for older people within the geographical area covered by each PCG. Participants included staff who planned or provided services, and older people and their carers who lived within the area. The localities were all within England and represented a broad range of socio-economic, geographical and health-related circumstances.

## Do older people want to be involved?

This study showed that older people and their carers (who are often old themselves) are interested in contributing their views and experience to help improve and develop services. People were keen to attend and interested in future events. The physical frailty and mental health problems that some older people experience need not prevent their involvement. Those who are unable to attend meetings can give their views in other ways, for example through discussion groups at day centres or interviews at home, hospital or care homes.

## What motivates older people to get involved?

PCGs and PCTs need to think carefully about the way they attract older people to get involved in service evaluation and planning, and need to understand something about what motivates older people to take part. Table 9.1 sets out the range of responses to telephone interviews with participants following the consultation events.

**Table 9.1** Reasons given for attending events and number of times each reason was given. (Some people gave more than one reason)

| Reasons given for attending consultation events | Total |
| --- | --- |
| To get information about services: | |
| to help me now and in future | 9 |
| to help other older people | 6 |
| to help me in the future | 1 |
| Because I have got experience of services | 9 |
| I wanted to give my views | 7 |
| I am interested in the subject | 6 |
| I wanted to hear other people's views/experiences | 5 |
| I like the person who invited me | 2 |
| Getting involved is part of being a responsible citizen | 2 |
| I hope others will benefit from my experience | 2 |
| If services improve I will benefit in the future | 1 |
| I wanted to find out more/see if I would be interested | 1 |
| I wanted to represent other users of the centre | 1 |
| For mental stimulation | 1 |

Organisations consulting older people often expressly invite the views of those they describe as 'service users' on the assumption that this is the best way to obtain views from people with direct experience of services. Thornton and Tozer (1995) found that older people who receive services may not identify themselves as 'users', particularly where this phrase implies either exploitation or dependency. Whilst professionals may relate to an individual as a service user, the individual may not see the services as central to life and therefore part of his or her identity. If older people are not well informed about what to expect from services or what is available, they will be disadvantaged in commenting on services. Improving information about services should go hand in hand with public involvement.

Those who participate may not believe that they will benefit directly from changes, but nevertheless wish to help others. In Table 9.1 a range of responses relates to benefits for other people. It is possible to appeal to these altruistic motives as a way to expand the scope of involvement. For example, older people can be recruited to undertake interviews, lead focus groups or conduct discussions with their peers.

# Attracting people

In most respects, older people will respond to invitations to get involved in a similar way to those in other age groups. It is possible to predict what is likely to work. Whether you are inviting older people to attend a consultation meeting, agree to be interviewed, join a focus group, complete a questionnaire or contribute to a working group, the same factors need to be considered.

- Describe the task clearly and show how it relates to the people invited. Older people are less often the focus of market research than younger age groups so the concepts and language about involvement may be less familiar.
- Describe the subject in a way that appeals to a range of motives, i.e. general interest in it, concern about outcome, citizens' responsibility, opportunity to influence the future.
- Any printed material needs to be as eye-catching as possible and in large print for people with visual impairments.
- Tell them how much time it will involve and consider convenience in terms of travel, timing and location. Many older people do not have access to a car; public transport may not be easy to use; some will have problems leaving home; some will prefer travelling in daylight.
- People will not expect to be out of pocket. You need to cover any costs. If they are giving a lot of time, a reward may be appropriate (in kind or cash).
- All contact (verbal, written and face-to-face) should be friendly, open and encourage contributions. Be aware of the impact of language, avoiding stereotypes about ageing and old age, or making assumptions about the audience. People should feel listened to and see evidence that their views are being recorded. Moreover, older people are more likely to have hearing impairment, so amplification or induction loops can help.
- If older people have to leave their homes to participate, the environment must be comfortable and user friendly, e.g. lighting, heat, access, refreshments, seating.
- In group situations, there should be lots of time to contribute, debate with others and share experiences. Older people attending the consultation events also enjoyed having enough time during breaks to talk informally with other participants.

- In one-to-one situations there needs to be time for clarification and to go at each person's pace.
- Tell them how their contributions will be used and how they will find out about the results.

## Involving older people and professionals together

The notion of users as consumers is strong in recent legislation and guidance, and implies that, for example, the dialogue between providers and users of social services is no different from that between a bank and its customers. However, as the literature indicates, these relationships are more complex. The way services are delivered can encourage those receiving services to believe that because they are not 'professional' they have no valid views on this subject (Owens and Batchelor, 1996). For example, if you believe that only a doctor is qualified to diagnose your health needs then you may decline from giving views, even on the non-medical aspects of the process of diagnosis.

Where people receive services from a particular individual, they are less likely to be critical of those services (Owens and Batchelor, 1996). This is thought to be partly due to a wish to avoid any retribution from the provider, but also because the personal relationship is valued even where the service is not entirely satisfactory. This may be an issue when people are being asked for views on services that are delivered on a one-to-one basis, for example single-handed GP services, practice nursing.

These findings indicate that consultation on personal health and social services is more complex than for some other types of service. Whilst guidance on consultation emphasises the value of direct dialogue between service providers and users, it is possible that this contact will prevent users expressing their real views and experiences. There are difficult choices to be made, such as whether users should be consulted without professionals being present. However, separate consultation rules out the possibility of discussion and clarification between the two parties; a significant problem if the issues are complex.

*Good idea to have a mix because professionals may see things differently from people who use services.*

In comparison to professionals, service users can be unintentionally disadvantaged by the way arrangements for involvement are made. In the events studied, it was harder for users to contribute when the discussion groups were large. Greater levels of formality often disadvantage users. Where some of the involvement is organised in small groups, the proportions of each group present during discussions can affect the outcome. Where users are in the minority they are less likely to express their views. Having a 50/50 balance, and experienced, well-briefed facilitators, will encourage everyone to contribute. Decisions about arrangements that appear to be insignificant can often have a large impact on participants.

> Having more professionals than older people on the group made it more difficult for me. I was worried about saying something silly.

Some of the older people invited to get involved will have had previous experience working in health or social care, and current experience in voluntary organisations providing related services. Similarly, professionals will have used some services and may also be carers. This can enrich the process as long as those organising activities are aware of the potential.

## Translating user views into service plans

Barnes and Walker (1996) suggest that users should not be expected to translate their experiences into formats that meet the needs of planners. It is the responsibility of those gathering information to analyse the views and experiences provided by users, and identify what the implications are in service terms.

There is increasing enthusiasm for 'whole systems' approaches to planning health and social services. If you ask older people and their carers about what works well for older people and what could be improved, they will tend to describe their experiences of the whole system. Due to their circumstances, they are most likely to be able to describe the gaps in services and to reflect on the importance of matters such as environment, transport and communication. At the events studied, the issues raised were mainly about community services that played a role in keeping people in their own homes. Issues that have a high media profile, such as 'trolley waits' in accident and emergency services, were rarely mentioned and not seen as priorities.

*Chemists hold my PIN and get my prescription, and they'll bring it for you.*

*Lifeline [personal emergency call system] is the one thing that allows me to stay at home.*

*There was no co-ordination. Why did the GP not know when the district nurse was visiting? I had expected a visit from the district nurse and she did not arrive. So I phoned my GP and asked if he knew where the district nurse was; he had no idea and no way to find out.*

Primary care is only one service area where statutory organisations are encouraged to involve users. All the partner organisations – community and acute trusts, health authorities and particularly social services – will be interested in making progress in this area. *The NHS Plan* (2000) makes it clear that the success of joint working between health and social services will be measured by how well they provide older people with improved services. PCGs and PCTs need to avoid duplicating the work of others and consider the greater impact that can be achieved through joint working. Older people, who have a keen interest in services being 'joined up', notice which organisations are represented at public events and on working groups.

## Building continuity and commitment

At each of the events, the older people placed a high priority on extending the ways in which they and their peers could be more involved locally. Their perception was that older people's voices were rarely heard or their opinions sought. The majority of those asked were also willing to participate in future consultation themselves.

Having invested resources in contact with some older people, it would make sense for PCGs and PCTs to try and maintain this contact. One-off events will not meet long-term planning needs or provide feedback on the quality of specific services. It is possible to maintain a group of people who can get involved in different ways over a longer period of time.

Local voluntary organisations may also have their own networks of users that could provide another source of involvement, for example Age Concern, Alzheimer's Disease Society. At practice level there are opportunities for involving older patients in service evaluation and development.

The challenge for primary care-based commissioners and providers of services is to understand how the whole system works and what could be done better. Older people and their carers are experts on the impact of services. They are enthusiastic partners in working to improve outcomes and will respond positively to invitations to get involved.

## References

Audit Commission. *The Coming of Age: improving care services for older people*. London: Audit Commission, 1997.

Barnes M, Walker A. Consumerism versus empowerment: a principled approach to the involvement of older service users, *Policy and Politics* 1996, vol. 24, no. 4: 375–94.

Department of Health. *The NHS Plan*. London: Department of Health, 2000.

Department of Social Security. *Building a Better Britain for Older People*. London: Department of Social Security, 1998.

Owens D, Batchelor C. Patient Satisfaction and the Elderly. *Social Science and Medicine* 1996; vol. 42, no. 11: 1483–91.

Thornton P, Tozer R. *Having a Say in Change*. York: Joseph Rowntree Foundation, 1995.

Chapter 10

# Patient involvement and clinical effectiveness

Brian Fisher and David Gilbert

## KEY POINTS

■ A local model is described whereby patients were engaged as teachers of primary care professionals in cardiac care and mental health.

■ Using patients as teachers has led to improvements in local health care delivery and changed professional behaviour.

■ Keys to success in the process included: being clear about objectives; identifying appropriate methodologies; and identifying the relevant stakeholders. This approach also helped build capacity for patient involvement among participants.

## Patient involvement and clinical effectiveness

In part, the rise of evidence-based practice can be viewed as a 'rationalist' or 'empiricist' movement predicated on the view that 'clinical decisions should be based on the best available scientific evidence' (Davidoff *et al.* 1995), rather than subjectivist notions of 'what works'. This approach does not necessarily include the needs and preferences of a range of patients who may hold different views about what constitutes 'evidence' and whose outcomes may not be represented in the research (Delamothe, 1999). Evidence-based practice often places knowledge in the hands of one set of 'experts' – the academic establishment. The 'hierarchy of evidence' can be seen as imposing a reductionist agenda across clinical practice. Since much research funding comes from commercial sources, clinical effectiveness can be seen as a way of concentrating power in the hands of doctors, academics and commercial interests, such as the pharmaceutical industry.

In contrast, there are a number of initiatives that seek to identify the things that matter to patients in terms of treatment outcomes (Kelson, 1999). These 'patient-centred outcomes' can also be incorporated into programmes of clinical audit (Kelson, 1998), effectiveness, clinical governance (Gilbert and Walker, 2000), or standard setting within National Service Frameworks.

This sort of work complements that undertaken in the field of shared decision-making: promoting individual patient choice by making evidence about the effectiveness of health care accessible to health service users, and the provision of high quality information (Coulter, Entwistle and Gilbert, 1998).

Patient involvement has been a feature of programmes to implement clinical effectiveness. 'Promoting Action on Clinical Effectiveness' (PACE) was a King's Fund programme that aimed to demonstrate the effective implementation of evidence-based practice. PACE used an integrated approach, based on a range of activities to change professional practice. Most of the 16 projects involved some element of patient involvement (Dunning *et al*. 1998).

Despite these initiatives, the precise role of patient involvement in clinical effectiveness is unclear to managers and clinicians alike. For many clinicians, patient involvement still means feeding patients information. This approach – whereby information moves from professional to patient – although valuable, reinforces existing power relationships.

We describe below a local approach to involving patients using a complementary model – with information flowing from patient to professional (see Figure 10.1). Clarifying patients' views of effectiveness and using these definitions productively is central. The key question to be asked of patients is 'What works for you?'

**Figure 10.1** An alternative model of patient involvement and clinical effectiveness

1. Patients informed about clinical effectiveness
professional          >>>          patient
(e.g. patient information materials, awareness-raising activities)

2. Patients informing clinical effectiveness development
professional          <<<          patient
(e.g. patients as agents of change)

Our experience suggests that patients can be involved in clinical effectiveness in the following ways:

- **at an individual level** – receiving information and acting as agents of change
- **at a collective level** – defining effectiveness and educating professionals.

## The LSL approach

Lambeth, Southwark and Lewisham Health Authority's 'Implementing Clinical Effectiveness' (ICE) programme supports primary care practices to do more of what is known to be effective, less of what is known to be ineffective, and to involve patients in the process.

The first stage is to identify three or four priority issues within a particular clinical area. The first area chosen in LSL was cardiac care, the second was mental health. An integrated approach to change in primary care was then designed. In cardiac care, this meant practices working with pharmacists, the Medical Audit Advisory Group (MAAG), practice nurses, health promotion teams and postgraduate educators. Guideline Amendment Groups developed and disseminated guidelines to local GPs and practice nurses. The service consequences of change for secondary care were planned and resourced. For example, finance for cardiac rehabilitation services and echocardiography was increased.

This multidimensional approach is a key mechanism for facilitating change in professional practice (Oxman *et al.* 1995). To make a difference, NSF implementation will need to incorporate these kinds of interventions.

## Patients as recipients of information

The simplest and most traditional method of involving patients is through the development and dissemination of patient information materials. Involving patients in the development of such materials is one means of improving their quality (Coulter, Entwistle and Gilbert, 1998).

Within mental health, an evidence-based booklet on depression was written by patients. Technical aspects, such as information about medication, were written by consultants. A list of questions users should ask of professionals is included in the booklet, adapted from the original developed by the Royal College of Psychiatrists. Piloted with local GPs, nurses and patients, it has been distributed to libraries, practices and pharmacists in LSL. Other methods of dissemination of clinical effectiveness information have included using the health authority's regular feature article in the south London press.

A co-ordinated dissemination strategy that targets both patients and the general public should not be seen as an 'add-on'. It requires a multi-disciplinary project team incorporating expertise such as writing and graphic design.

## Patients as change agents

In the fields of HIV and obstetrics, for example, patient power has been a significant force for change. By providing patients with the same clinical effectiveness information that professionals receive, patients may stimulate professionals to improve their quality of care (Rosser, McDowell and Newell, 1991). This trend is being reinforced by developments in information technology. More and more, this means that professionals will have to become 'navigators for patients' through increasing amounts of information, and not merely 'providers' of care and knowledge.

Although this approach remains at an early stage in LSL, the ICE programme has translated its GP guidelines into lay versions that provide essentially the same information to patients. The leaflet on depression encourages questioning on the part of the user.

## Patients as definers of effectiveness

Those leading the ICE programme recognised the importance of empowering patients at the individual level, but they also wanted to do more to allow the lay voice to influence collective service delivery and planning. Qualitative methodologies were used to investigate patients' own views on what works well for them. In the cardiac work, eight patients discussed their experiences of cardiac care and about 'what worked'. The discussion was analysed and generated the following themes:

**Information** – There was a strong desire for comprehensive information covering the nature of the illness, its severity and planned treatment. Practical information was sought on services (e.g. out-patient appointments and investigation results) and how to cope with the illness.

**Dignity and respect** – Patients should be treated as equals. The group saw patients as having a role in prompting medical staff and in indicating what patients wanted to know. Medical staff should understand and appreciate the patient's perspective and offer information in ways that match the patient's values and capabilities. Respect and politeness made difficult times better.

**After-care** – Support in the month following discharge from hospital was seen as very important. This aspect of the recovery process was considered frightening, as support systems seemed to 'disappear' and lack of co-ordination between primary and secondary care became apparent. For example, there were stories about repeat prescriptions not being provided before medication ran out, questions about care and treatment not being answered, and emergencies not being defined so that untoward events were interpreted as crises.

Though there is a dearth of literature that examines the experiences of cardiac patients in any detail, there is some evidence that validates these experiences (Thompson, Ersser and Webster, 1995). Meeting information needs is associated positively with cardiac patients' satisfaction (Larson, Nelson, Gustafson and Batalden, 1996).

These conclusions were incorporated into ICE guidelines that went out to every GP and practice nurse in LSL. The findings prompted LSL HA and the PACE programme to fund a cardiac nurse to support patients in the first month after returning home, and to help local practices in providing effective cardiac management and better linking with secondary care.

## Patients as teachers

In LSL, patients have begun to teach primary care professionals about effective practice. This builds on work being done elsewhere on patients delivering professional education programmes, educating professionals about aspects of long-term illness, and using 'expert patients' to aid other patients in self-help for their condition (Carr *et al.* 1999; Graley, Nettle and Wallcraft, 1994).

Whereas the 'expert patient' programme is primarily designed to empower patients to manage their own condition, the 'patients as teachers' process also aims to educate professionals about how they should care for and treat patients.

The aims of the process are to:

- identify effective clinical interventions as defined by users
- use these as teaching tools for practice staff
- investigate the acceptability of this process for participants
- assess the impact of the intervention
- develop a set of user-defined outcome measures
- incorporate outcomes into local policy.

## Patients as teachers in cardiac care

Put simply, the 'patients as teachers' process involves delegates from patient focus groups meeting professionals to discuss 'what works' from their own point of view. The process has been carried out in cardiac care and mental health, and is planned to be taken forward with young people who have asthma. Here, we describe the process and outcomes in cardiac care for which there is the most thorough data.

Four focus groups of patients were recruited: one of women (mixed ages), one of men (under 65), one of older people (mixed gender, over 65 years), and one group of people from the Asian community. This cross-section of groups was chosen to represent patient populations where there is evidence that they have differences in clinical presentation and outcomes. The groups were professionally facilitated, and discussions were taped, transcribed and analysed.

The groups were asked: 'In your experience, what has worked best for you in the management of your heart disease?' This approach was designed to elicit constructive comment on the quality of care. Self-selected delegates from the groups then met with primary care clinicians – 20 GPs and six nurses – in two professionally facilitated (PGEA accredited) meetings. Professionals were encouraged to listen and be receptive to patients' views. Feedback from the focus groups and recommendations from the meetings were provided to each participant.

## Patients' recommendations

There were two main sets of recommendations that came from patients: first, those to do with practitioners' delivery of care and treatment; second, those concerning organisational issues. With regard to the former, issues raised included information provision and 'consultation style'. An effective practitioner, according to patients, provided timely and appropriate information. Patients did not want to be patronised, and valued being treated with respect and dignity. The involvement of relatives was also recommended.

The following practice management issues were highlighted:

- clinicians should bar telephone interruptions during consultations
- flexible appointment systems – with appointments of different durations according to need – were requested
- people wanted clear and efficient processes by which they received test results, with more information provided about their meaning
- regular follow-ups would be helpful
- better use could be made of telephone contacts.

## Professional change

The professional participants were surveyed after six months and asked about what changes they had implemented as a result of the meeting (see Table 10.1). Substantial change was reported in relation to many patient recommendations, including involvement in treatment decisions (e.g. through provision of information), practice management issues (e.g. reducing phone interruptions, offering flexible appointment lengths) and continuity of care (e.g. referrals to rehabilitation care). The issue of investigation results was taken up by one local PCG as part of its clinical governance initiatives.

**Table 10.1** Professional change after six months

### Recommendations put into practice
*(Percentage of participants saying they had implemented these changes since meeting with patient delegates – note small sample size, n=20)*

| | |
|---|---|
| Using videos | 13% |
| Providing more information to patients about side effects | 80% |
| Providing leaflets to patients | 66% |
| Developing/enhancing system for providing test results | 60% |
| Developing/enhancing system for regular reviews | 47% |
| Providing interpreters | 53% |
| Increasing referrals to cardiac rehab | 40% |
| Providing Medic-Alert bracelets | 7% |
| Involving families more | 60% |
| Reducing phone interruptions | 53% |
| Offering appointments of different lengths | 60% |

### Aspects of consultation style changed since group

| | |
|---|---|
| Trying to find out what patient most wants to know | 60% |
| Offering more information about the illness | 53% |
| Asking 'What do you most want information about?' | 33% |
| Offering more information about medication | 53% |
| Offering more information about investigations | 60% |

When compared to other educational interventions that show little effect in terms of professional change (Davis, Thomson, Oxman and Haynes, 1995), it appears that this patient-mediated intervention has a positive impact on practice. The precise drivers for change warrant further investigation. The 'face-to-face' aspect may be significant, as may the credibility of the testimony provided by 'real' patients.

Participants appreciated the process. All patients found the meetings interesting and useful. Most gained new information from the meetings. None found them frightening or felt there were issues that they could not raise. Patients' views on effective practice seem, according to those who took part, to be useful, precise and appropriate, with suggestions involving specific changes in practice organisation. The overall cost was approximately £11,000.

## Patients as teachers in mental health

The process has been repeated in mental health, the second ICE topic in LSL. Four focus groups were convened with users of mental health services, each comprising a separate category of user: the first had been diagnosed with psychosis; the second, with severe depression; the third, with moderate depression; and the fourth was an ethnic minority group with illness defined as 'moderate'.

## Patient recommendations

The major recommendations arising were as follows:

**Access and continuity** – People wanted easier access to a GP. GPs need to grasp when patients are having difficulties, to be clear about their own limitations, and to know when to refer patients on to other parts of the service. Continuity of care is of prime importance.

**Communication** – Users appreciated empathetic practitioners who were able to deal with a crisis calmly and recognise that mental pain can be very distressing. In terms of 'probing' at problems, they need to do this gently. People may not want to 'open up' until they are ready. Clinicians need to be able to communicate clearly when a consultation is at an end, rather than merely appearing irritable.

**Outside the consultation** – Receptionists also need to have more understanding of mental health problems. Privacy is important – many patients would prefer to wait in a quiet part of the waiting room.

## Professional change

A qualitative study (Cranfield, 2000) of GPs' and nurses' reactions to the patient–professional seminar on mental health contacted 62 per cent of participants. The following changes had taken place as a result of the intervention:

- more tolerance for patients' behaviour in the waiting room
- health checks were offered for patients with mental illness
- prioritising of mental health training for reception staff
- development of a methadone prescribing service
- development of a user group
- improvements to the appointment system.

The process was seen as meaningful and had an impact on participants' perspectives on mental health problems. There was some concern that patients at the joint meeting seemed to find it difficult to act as representatives rather than as individuals with their own stories that needed to be told.

## Implications

While there is some evidence that involving patients in their own care and treatment can improve outcomes, there has been little evaluation of the way in which a collective patient voice can influence efforts to improve service quality. The LSL HA approach to involving patients in its clinical effectiveness programme has gone some way towards bridging this gap.

## Outcomes

Many of the recommendations made by patients accord with similar work carried out elsewhere. For example, recent work at the Princess Alexandra Hospital NHS Trust confirms the importance of access and continuity issues for cardiac patients across secondary and primary care (e.g. discharge arrangements or 'coming home') (Gilbert and Walker, 2000). The recent public consultation on *The NHS Plan* highlighted similar issues of importance to patients, such as the clinical and human aspects of care, the environment of care, promotion of health, and access and continuity issues (Office for Public Management, 2000).

The LSL approach appears to have had an effect on changing professional behaviour and has helped local organisations to incorporate patient-centred outcomes in their work. It has provided a practical, cost-effective intervention to improve quality and empower patients.

## Practical issues

The 'patients as teachers' process is generalisable across different contexts and clinical areas. It might be used as part of clinical effectiveness programmes, clinical governance or joint agency approaches, such as Health Improvement Programmes (as has been done in LSL). Such approaches may be supported by PCGs. Although ICE covered the health authority, the intimacy of PCGs may make similar work easier to incorporate in clinical practice.

As patients become involved in the process, they become more informed. Delegates learn to represent the collective voice rather than merely talk about their own stories. Organisations struggling with how to involve 'real' patients and move beyond engaging the 'usual suspects' can use the process to engage in constructive dialogue with their client groups. However, this requires organisations to support patients (with resources, training and administrative back-up) so that they can do the job well. Those involved in the process can become part of patient forums or other structures required of organisations in *The NHS Plan*.

Keys to success in the process include being clear about aims and objectives, identifying appropriate methodologies, and identifying the relevant stakeholders. Building capacity for patient involvement – finding ways of supporting patients and professionals, so that the former can contribute properly and the latter can be receptive enough to respond properly – is also vital.

## Changing professional culture

The LSL approach seems to be a safe and effective way of promoting dialogue between patients and professionals, but it does pose some challenges to traditional power relationships.

The 'patients as teachers' process illustrates that there are often mutually agreed ways forward to deal with problems amongst patients and professionals. The 'value-added' benefit of patient involvement is that it can provide a practical perspective on problems and solutions. The force of individual patient testimony can also be a powerful trigger for individuals to change.

Sackett has proposed a model of evidence-based practice that does not imply such a confrontation of knowledge systems (Sackett, 1996). He suggests that the arenas of evidence-based practice, clinical competence and patient preferences are overlapping circles of influence, each representing a valid knowledge system. The LSL approach suggests a feasible model for incorporating these concepts into day-to-day work.

Many fears surrounding patient involvement have arisen because mechanisms for engaging patients in decision-making have been lacking. In the absence of such mechanisms, patient views are marginalised, professionals make false assumptions about what patients need, organisations come to distrust 'outspoken' patient representatives, and polarisation between local communities and NHS organisations prevails. Processes such as those described above can help to overcome these problems, build dialogue and aid understanding. Most importantly, they can help to improve patient care.

## References

Coulter A, Entwistle V, Gilbert D. *Informing patients: an assessment of the quality of patient information materials*. London: King's Fund, 1998.

Cranfield S. *Listening to Patients Health First*. London: Lambeth Southwark and Lewisham Health Authority, August 2000.

Davidoff *et al*. Evidence based medicine. A new journal to help doctors identify the information they need. BMJ 1995; 310: 1085–86.

Davis D A, Thomson M A, Oxman A D, Haynes B. Changing Physician Performance: a systematic review of the effect of continuing medical education strategies. JAMA 1995; vol. 274, no. 9.

Delamothe T. Using outcomes research in clinical practice. Editorial. BMJ 1994; 308: 1583–84.

Dunning M, Abi-Aad G, Gilbert D, Hutton H, Brown C. *Experience, Evidence and Everyday Practice*. London: King's Fund, 1999.

Gilbert D, Walker M. *Involving patients in clinical governance*. London: Office for Public Management and the Princess Alexandra Hospital NHS Trust, 2000.

Kelson M. *Patient defined outcomes*. London: College of Health, 1999.

Kelson M. *Promoting patient involvement in clinical audit: Practical guidance on achieving effective involvement*. London: College of Health, 1998.

Larson C O, Nelson E C, Gustafson D, Batalden P B. The relationship between meeting patients' information needs and their satisfaction with hospital care and general health status outcomes. *Int. Jl. for Qual. in Hlth. Care* 1996; 8 (5): 447–56.

Office for Public Management. *Shifting Gears. Report of the public consultation on the NHS Plan*. London: 2000.

Oxman A *et al*. No magic bullets: a systematic review of 102 trials of interventions to improve general practice. *CMAJ* 1995; 153: 1423–31.

Rosser W W, McDowell I, Newell C. Use of reminders for preventative procedures in family medicine. *CMAJ* 1991; 145: 807–14.

Sackett D L *et al*. Evidence based medicine: what it is and what it isn't. *BMJ* 1996; 312: 71–72.

Chapter 11

# Community development in primary care

Brian Fisher

---

### KEY POINTS

- Community development is an effective means for primary care organisations to respond to the challenges of public involvement and health inequalities.

- Health professionals and their organisations need training and support to work productively with the public as partners.

- The NHS needs to work with community development organisations to move from consultation to participation.

- The Government, which declares its commitment to public participation, needs to offer a clearer agenda and more support in order to encourage the process.

---

## Introduction

*Inclusionary policies are those which enhance the social, economic and political power of groups in subordinate positions in society; in short, they promote the autonomy of marginal groups.* (Farrar, 1996)

The interaction between GP and patient is a small part of the mesh of influences that determines the course of the patient's health. Beyond that brief exchange lies the community and the social forces that foster or hinder health.

The Labour government has understood this in attempting to address the wider determinants of ill health (Department of Health, 1997; Department of Health, 1998) and has recommended a range of responses of varying practicability. In addition, communities are seen as a key level at which users of health services can become involved in local health care planning and delivery (NHS Executive, 2000). *The NHS Plan* embraces the national strategy for neighbourhood renewal, plans for health visitors and community nurses to work with local communities to improve health, and a Healthy Communities Collaborative to spread best practice (Allen, 2000). Against a background of many years promoting community development in Lewisham, what does the concept have to offer primary care professionals and the people they serve?

## Definition

Community health development is a process by which people are involved in collectively defining and taking action on issues that affect their health. The community sets the agenda and work is usually with groups rather than individuals (Barker, Bullen and de Ville, 1999).

The term 'community' requires its own definition. A community can be seen as a group of people who have something in common. Two types can be distinguished, and work with each will have different characteristics:

- **a geographic community** is a group of people who live in the same area. This may be a housing estate, for instance, with people using the same shops and services. It is not necessarily an electoral ward, which may consist of a number of different groups who feel they live in different areas with different needs. These distinctions are particularly important in the inner city.
- **a community of interest** is a social group that shares particular characteristics, but may not share geography, e.g. people with heart disease or people from a minority ethnic group.

It may also be helpful to distinguish between the terms 'consultation' and 'participation' (Fisher, 1994):

- **consultation** can be seen as viewing the public as consumers in order to receive information and advice from them.
- **participation** can be seen as involvement of the public as partners in order to service or empower them where they have expanded power and control.

The Lewisham Community Development Partnership (LCDP) (Kawachi and Kennedy, 1997) a health project in south-east London (see below), describes its work as having three components:

- listening to local people's needs and recommendations for health improvement as described by them
- working with local people to implement those recommendations
- providing services, defined and designed by local communities.

In the next section, we examine the outcomes that can be expected from community development, as well as examples of good practice.

## The benefits of community development

There are good reasons for this interest in community development. There are examples of its usefulness at a number of levels in the NHS and elsewhere, and a number of such projects have been chosen as Beacon sites. The main benefits include:

- **improving networks in a community**. This process has been shown to have a protective effect on health (Berkman and Syme, 1979).
- **identifying health needs from the users' points of view**, in particular those of marginalised groups and those suffering health inequalities.
- **change and influence**. Supporting the participation of local people in improving their own health enhances local planning and delivery of health services.
- **developing local services and structures that act as a resource**. These can often be preventive, for instance playgrounds run with the involvement of children, providing alternatives for kids who would otherwise be at risk of violence or accidents.
- **improving self-esteem and learning new skills that can aid employment** by becoming involved in community activities.
- **widening the boundaries of the health debate by involving people in defining their views on health and local services**. Here, issues of local relevance become apparent, e.g. housing, education. An inter-agency strategy becomes more likely.
- **tackling underlying causes of ill health and disadvantage** with greater likelihood of success.

There is now an increasing body of literature which shows that being part of a social network of contacts, whether it be church, friends and relations, or groups and activities, is protective for health (Hemingway and Marmot, 1999). This effect is surprisingly powerful and it seems to extend across a number of clinical modalities, including heart disease (Pennix, van Tilberg, Kriegsman *et al.* 1997) and the problems of older people (Lewisham Community Development Partnership, 1998). These effects are probably mediated through improved self-esteem, trust and increased feelings of being in control. These aspects of group involvement are sometimes described as 'social capital'. A simple example of this kind of work might be reminiscence groups for more active older people or family food groups (Crowley, 1997).

---

**Norwich Community Health Partnership Food Group**

The group cooks (and eats!) healthy food, affordable for people on a low income. Their confidence in cooking has increased. The group provided the impetus for many other activities, for instance providing cooking lessons in a local school, developing a hygiene course, and planning a community café.

---

By asking local people about the health issues that matter to them, very clear recommendations for health planners can be defined. By pursuing these ideas collectively, implementation is more likely. The Newcastle experience has shown that organising large-scale meetings between local people and health managers can be very effective at producing change (Murray and Graham, 1995).

---

**Community Action on Health, Newcastle**

A number of existing groups were brought together with local GPs and the health authority, while work was co-ordinated with local people on an individual basis. These disparate groups are brought together once a year, having concentrated in the previous year on a range of issues defined as relevant by residents. Their recommendations have been included in commissioning plans.

Community development approaches are effective as needs assessment. They often eschew dealing with established voluntary organisations that may have their own agendas to pursue. There is some evidence that the more involved the community is in needs assessment, the more likely changes are to ensue (Gillam and Murray, 1996). Community development seeks to involve those who are least engaged with existing services or structures. Because traditional community workers use eclectic methods, including work on estates, working in pubs and clubs, as well as questionnaires and focus groups, community development can tap into groups and areas of concern and interest that are otherwise difficult to access. Such methods can reach people who are unlikely to attend neighbourhood forums or public meetings.

---

**Lewisham's Youth Health Advisor**

One example of this process operating successfully is the development of the Youth Health Advisor post in south-east London. A summer playscheme organised by the LCDP discussed health issues with the children involved. They made a series of recommendations for improvements that included changes to consultation style as well as the development of a new post. These observations were checked with a survey, designed by the public health department of the health authority, across local schools and youth clubs. This person would not only involve young people in their own health education, but also act as an advocate for them with local practices. Funding for this post was agreed and evaluation has shown beneficial educational outcomes for young people and professionals.

---

Many community development projects develop local services that did not previously exist in the locality. They can be very effective if well targeted and organised. An example is an initiative in Belfast, defined and designed by local people (Popay and Williams, 1996).

**Opportunity Youth in Belfast**
Working with young people as peer educators, exciting work has been done with 300 disadvantaged youths. Activities include heightening awareness of statutory services, individual counselling, an antenatal programme, and health awareness groups, including work on drugs and sex education. Evaluation showed that employment prospects improved as a result of the intervention.

Because lay people have different health beliefs to professionals, their approach to improvements in health care are different and often take a wider perspective. For instance, they will readily identify issues of transport, housing, education and stress as important mechanisms that can lead to poor health for themselves and their families (Laughlin and Black, 1995). This encourages an inter-agency approach.

**The Lewisham Bus**
Sydenham is a hilly area, and local GPs were having to respond to elderly patients with chronic obstructive pulmonary disease struggling to the shops. The community worker, having consulted local people, suggested a new bus route to alleviate the problem. As a result of negotiation with the local authority, this has now been successfully in operation for some years.

Insofar as tackling poverty is concerned, a survey examined 100 projects on poverty and health (Henderson, 1997). This noted that a range of benefits had accrued to participants. These included increasing income for individuals and communities, improving the quality of life in communities, and providing better services such as mental health. In addition, healthy lifestyles to prevent coronary heart disease had been promoted, and there were practical results of campaigning, such as housing improvements and play areas.

> **The Vrieheide Project**
> The neighbourhood of Vrieheide in the Netherlands had all the characteristics of the run-down inner city. Community workers and residents worked together to combat criminality, improving school conditions and supporting initiatives that reduced unemployment. Success was the result of concentrating on existing problems of the residents, dealing with small-scale issues, excellent communication and publicity.

## The limitations of community development

Many of the problems raised by community development stem from its strengths. This approach is not a quick fix. A community development organisation cannot simply be grafted onto an existing structure with swift results. The process takes time to become embedded in a community for trust and understanding to build on both sides.

Outcomes can be unpredictable. The consultation process, with responses from local people, is not always a comfortable one. Because the issues raised often imply multi-agency responses, they may be more difficult, and possibly more expensive, to respond to.

Evaluation can be difficult as the inputs are complex and often best described in qualitative terms. Nonetheless, evaluation is possible, and a valuable King's Fund guide offers a range of useful techniques (Freeman *et al.* 1997).

Community development workers often come from outside the NHS family. Their voluntary sector or local authority roots can sit uneasily within primary care organisations. Mutual learning takes time and commitment.

## Community development work at practice level – successes and stresses

There is increasing experience of this relationship which, despite conflicts and insecurities, can be very productive. Community development is most commonly used to carry out a needs assessment of either a representative proportion of the practice population, or a particular population, such as drug users. This has been used to discuss issues within a practice and to define ways of implementing change. Examples of outcomes of this process include changes in appointment systems, times of practice opening, improved liaison with the housing department, as well as changes in consultation technique.

The advantage of this approach is that practice members, who would otherwise be unlikely to participate in such an activity, can listen to their patients with minimal time commitment and in an environment that is safe for the professionals. A number of PCG/Ts are using this approach as part of their user involvement strategy.

However, as with all such processes, there are strains in the system. What if users 'ask for the moon'? How do you deal with the onslaught of complaints and problems that might arise, not to mention the disappointment of patients whose demands are rejected?

Our experience in Lewisham is reassuring. First, patients are only too well aware of the strains in the system. They are usually reluctant to make difficult or expensive demands. Second, the requests and recommendations are frequently about the approach of the practice as a whole. That is, they tend to be concerned with system issues such as consultation style or organisational changes. Although these may be difficult to respond to, they are rarely threatening to the organisation or the individuals within it, and they are not usually expensive to change. Third, where requests are problematic, most practices have found compromise solutions that are satisfactory. Fourth, the practice retains the right to refuse.

## Support for professionals in responding to user views

This is not to suggest that listening and responding to users' views carries no threat to health professionals and managers. This is far from the case. Our experience shows that practice members are liable to conflate a number of related 'dangers':

- hearing recommendations for a change in approach is equivalent to receiving a complaint

- a complaint is experienced as a personal attack
- users are likely to ask for expensive items, items that they are unlikely to be able (or want) to respond to
- start discussions and the 'floodgates will open' – they will lose control of the practice entirely
- patients are 'loose cannons' – there's no predicting where this process will lead
- listening to patients' wants is a poor basis for making changes to systems that have been developed over years.

It is not sufficient to exhort health professionals with the adage that 'every complaint is a treasure' when the structure of general practice encourages an entrepreneurial and personal approach to delivering care. The distinctions between consultation and participation need to be made clearer to many health professionals.

In addition, there are organisational restrictions: practices are often static structures, with systems geared more to staff than patient needs. It can be difficult to see the necessity for change and it can be difficult to implement it, even if the need is agreed. More meetings, more time – these are serious disincentives in an overstretched system.

Critical Incident Analysis or Significant Event Monitoring within clinical governance provides a platform on which may be built more robust and supportive programmes to encourage and explore these issues. Although the Government's thrust is primarily to guard against interventions that are a threat to health, clinical governance needs to be expanded to integrate complaints and user involvement strategies. Personal Medical Services (PMS) pilots provide another vehicle for innovation; for example, user involvement is included as an element in PMS contracts.

## Community development at PCG/T level

Whether the development of more locally focused organisations such as PCTs will actually foster the effective use of these techniques, and the use of the information and energy they can deliver, remains to be seen. So far, PCG/Ts have not rated user involvement very highly. Among a long list of 'must dos' this comes low on their list of priorities (Anderson and Florin, 2000). Across the country, community development is increasingly seen as a useful mechanism for accessing the views of local people, but PCG involvement remains patchy (Anderson, 2000).

One example of how community development is slowly becoming integrated into PCG/T work is in Lewisham, south-east London. Here, two neighbouring PCGs are working with the same community development organisation, Lewisham Community Development Partnership (LCDP), to carry out a number of functions.

First, the organisation is working with a number of neighbouring single-handed practices to consult with their patients and develop a set of recommendations for improvement. All the practices have undertaken to listen and respond to the feedback. It seems clear that patients of these practices have a high rate of satisfaction with the service they receive, valuing their accessibility and continuity. Second, there are a number of services provided by the organisation that are actively used by local people and practices. These include a health library, a summer playscheme, a counselling service, and a football league bringing local disaffected youth together. Third, the PCG has responded to a needs assessment carried out by LCDP on the housebound elderly (Lewisham Community Development Partnership, 1999) in its strategy for older people. Findings included isolation, low satisfaction with social service provision, a need for better provision of aids and adaptations, and an appreciation of the problems caused by the health and social services divide. Fourth, the findings from a survey of the needs of mental health users (Wilson and Gill, 1999) have been incorporated into local mental health strategy. Users' views are therefore being reflected in planning.

Producing data is rarely sufficient to ensure change. Community development may be more effective than more abstract methods at bringing the concerns of local people to the attention of those with the power to make changes. By combining representative information with the force of local voices, it is more likely that their recommendations will be taken seriously. Nonetheless, there is more work to be done encouraging both professionals and voluntary organisations to engage with the public in a participatory rather than consultative manner.

PCTs' lay boards will not guarantee responsiveness to local people, as experience with health authorities has shown. It will be necessary to ensure that there are coherent and effective structures within the PCT that can deliver on public involvement in general and community development in particular (see Chapter 3).

In addition, government support is essential to move this process along. The lack of identified funding and development work for user involvement has hindered its development at local level. The successes described above are the result of enlightened health authorities and local authorities, and a fortunate concatenation of organisations and circumstances. What is needed now is the integration of project work into mainstream thinking and service delivery.

The Government's commitment to health visitors and district nurses working with local communities is a welcome step, but may not be enough. It is unlikely that these professionals will have the time or the skills to carry out this kind of work; it will remain a marginal aspect of their work. Community workers have a long tradition of working in an eclectic way with a wide range of groups and ensuring that professionals stay 'on tap, but not on top'; it will be difficult for health professionals to learn these techniques. In addition, as GPs have found, there may be an inherent contradiction between the ethos of working individually and that of working collectively for the local population.

## Conclusion

Community development is a well-recognised and effective means for involving the public and users in health issues. Community development can also be an important resource for the PCT to respond to the social forces that have a more profound effect on health than the health service itself. It is beginning to be employed in primary care to develop services and to integrate user views into planning. PCTs offer an opportunity to take community development forward, but it will need continuing support from government. Practices need education on how to engage with users, enhancing the Critical Incident Analysis process. They have incentives to put this learning into practice. The same is required at the level of the PCG/T board.

# References

Allen P. Accountability for clinical governance: developing collective responsibility for quality in primary care. *BMJ* 2000; 321: 608–11.

Anderson P. *Tackling health inequalities – is it a bridge too far for PCGs?* Primary Care Report, Sept 2000.

Anderson W, Florin D. *Involving the Public – one of many priorities.* London: King's Fund, 2000.

Barker J, Bullen M, de Ville J. *Reference Manual for Public Involvement.* London: South Bank University, 2000.

Berkman L F, Syme S L. Social networks, host resistance and mortality: a nine-year follow-up of Alameda County residents. *Am. J. Epidemiol.* 1979; 109: 186–204.

Community Health Development. *An evaluation of work in Mile Cross and Catton Grove, Norwich, 1993–5.* Norwich: Norwich Community Health Partnership NHS Trust.

Crowley P. *Community Action on Health. Annual Report 1997.* Newcastle: West End Resource, 1997.

Department of Health. *Shared Contributions, Shared Benefits: the report of the working group on public health and primary care.* London: Department of Health, 1997.

Department of Health. *Our Healthier Nation – a contract for health.* London: Department of Health, 1998; Cm 3852.

Farrar M. Black communities and processes of exclusion. In: Haughton G, Williams C C, editors. *Corporate City?* Aldershot: Avebury, 1996.

Fisher B, Neve H, Heritage Z. Community development, user involvement and primary care. *BMJ* 1999; 318: 749–50.

Fisher B. The Wells Park Health Project. In: Heritage Z, editor. *Community Participation in Primary Care.* London: Royal College of General Practitioners, 1994.

Freeman R, Gillam S, Shearin C, Pratt J. *Community Development and Involvement in Primary Care.* London: King's Fund, 1997.

Gilllam S, Murray S. *Needs Assessment in General Practice.* Occasional Paper 73. London: Royal College of General Practitioners, 1996.

Hemingway H, Marmot M. Psychosocial factors in the aetiology and prognosis of coronary heart disease: systematic review of prospective cohort studies. *BMJ* 1999; 318: 1460–67.

Kawachi I, Kennedy B P. Health and social cohesion: why care about income inequality? *BMJ* 1997; 314: 1037–40.

Laughlin S, Black D, editors. *Poverty and Health: Tools for Change: Ideas, analysis, information, action.* Birmingham: The Public Health Alliance, 1995.

Murray S, Graham L. Practice-based needs assessment: use of four methods in a small neighbourhood. *BMJ* 1995; 310: 1443–48.

NHS Executive. *The NHS Plan. A plan for investment. A plan for reform.* Cm 4818–I. London: The Stationery Office, 2000.

Pennix B, van Tilberg T, Kriegsman D *et al.* Effects of social support and personal coping resources on mortality in older age: the Longitudinal Ageing Study Amsterdam. *Am. J. Epidemiol.* 1997; 146: 510–19.

Popay J, Williams G. Public health and lay knowledge. *Soc. Sci. Med.* 1996; 311: 42–50.

Wilson M, Gill S. *Primary Care Mental Health. Assessing Users' Needs – the Sydenham Locality Project.* A MIND/LCDP collaboration, 1999.

# Conclusions

Fiona Brooks and Stephen Gillam

## Context

This book set out to explore the value of public and patient involvement in primary care. The contributions have pointed to central challenges facing managers and health professionals in grappling with the challenges of user involvement. The book may also assist service users to understand the nature of change required in the organisational and professional culture of primary care. The central challenges identified in the text are:

- **A policy environment** in which the NHS is required to become more responsive to the needs and preferences of users and carers, and where a new range of bodies and services are being put in place enabling their voices to be heard (NHS Executive, 2000). Separately, efforts are being made to speed up access to services in ways that may undermine traditional professional–patient relationships. Many health professionals feel threatened by these developments and may resist engaging with the Government's modernisation agenda.
- **Organisational changes** that are placing huge pressures on health professionals, requiring them to play a greater part in management and in running health organisations, while also working directly with patients. The advent of new primary care organisations and new partnerships with social care offer exciting opportunities for all parties, but they may also distract from the business of improving the way individual practitioners engage with patients.
- **Professional developments** that increasingly determine and restrict what individual practitioners may do. Protocols, guidelines and National Service Frameworks should reduce variations in performance and promote good practice, but they also constrain professional autonomy and may impede shared decision-making between professionals and patients. Increasing recognition of the need to integrate care across professional, organisational and sectoral boundaries means that a wide range of professionals (doctors, nurses, therapists, social workers and others) have to co-operate and ensure

continuity of care as the individual moves through the health and social care system. In these circumstances, both professionals and patients have to negotiate with a number of people as decisions are made over periods of time. The one-off consultation between practitioner and patient is therefore only one aspect of a complex pattern of relationships.

The drive towards user involvement can too easily be seen as a threat that will overwhelm primary care professionals through increasing demand combined with bureaucratic constraints. Alternatively, user involvement represents a means to meet the central challenge facing the health service: of managing competing demands and of improving its effectiveness (Slowie, 1999). Five key themes have threaded through the chapters in this book as central issues underpinning user involvement in primary health care. For primary health care to provide users with an effective voice in health care decision-making and service planning, progress in these five areas will be a prerequisite.

## 1. Shared values

Initiatives to improve the quality of services need to start from the perspective of the user and the context of users' lives, not professional or organisational needs (Wright, 1999; Beresford et al. 2000). At the level of the consultation, the concept of 'patient-centred medicine' has focused on the nature of shared decision-making. The case studies testify to patients' expertise and their capacity to make informed or evidence-based choices.

This change is of central importance if an antagonistic relationship between providers and users is to be avoided, because at the heart of many criticisms of the health service is the notion of a 'democratic deficit'. Popular though the health service remains, this particular arm of the Welfare State has come under increasing criticism for its lack of accountability. In this respect, as several contributors suggest, user involvement is of value in itself.

To achieve an accountable service will require a change in the cultural response from providers to challenges to professional authority, real or implied. (The Expert Patients Task Force, promoting lay-led approaches to the self-management of chronic conditions as part of *Saving Lives: Our Healthier Nation*, is one indication of genuine change at the centre (Department of Health, 2000).) This means that professionals will need to value and nurture the development of critical and well-informed users/citizens/stakeholders. However, accepting the responsibility for decision-making can be a daunting prospect for both users and providers.

As the opening chapter demonstrated, the public's priorities are not value free (Bowling, 1996; Stronks *et al.* 1997). There is merit in a shared set of ethical principles for those involved in making decisions about health care. The Tavistock Group has published a working draft for just such a framework, within which all stakeholders, including users of health services, can consider competing priorities (Smith *et al.* 1999).

## 2. Clarity of purpose

As we have seen, user involvement in primary care is hardly new. However, the increasing volume of rhetoric in this area has intensified pressure to demonstrate progress in what will ever be difficult territory. In such a situation, if user involvement is to be effective and sustainable, it is essential to retain clarity about the purpose of user involvement, target audiences, methods and desired outcomes (Barnes and Wistow, 1992).

For primary care organisations, these purposes may embrace assessing health and service needs to inform strategy development, establishing investment priorities and seeking feedback on quality. These aims are paralleled at the level of the individual clinical encounter: assessing individual needs, agreeing approaches to management and reviewing progress. The ultimate aim is, of course, to improve health, but too much public involvement is poorly co-ordinated. It takes time to develop ownership of this agenda across a practice or Primary Care Group. Early successes will help sustain interest. However, strategies that pay lip-service to user participation – through simplistic consultation or representation without sharing feedback, action or power – are not only unethical but damaging. A constant refrain, for example among representatives of black and minority ethnic communities, is that they are 'fed up' with needs assessment exercises that yield no obvious service changes. The phrase 'needs addressment' captures the importance of ensuring linkage at the outset between the processes of assessment and action (Brambleby, 2000).

## 3. The need for adequate resources

PCG/T boards may underestimate the organisational development required to involve users effectively. This work is time-consuming, requiring particular skills and commitment. It also requires a budget. On the other hand, health professionals and managers starting out have often exaggerated fears of being overwhelmed by user demands.

The selection of partners can be difficult, and Levenson has warned against 'Catch 23' (Levenson, 2000). This is the notion that anyone able to be involved in health and social care is not representative by definition. User involvement must embrace excluded groups but should not exclude those willing to do work with statutory organisations. The latter should be challenged to spread the net more widely to attract others: in other words, to avoid the 'usual suspect syndrome' but not to apply standards to lay people that would not be applied to others ('Who do you represent exactly?'). Creative public involvment is not guaranteed by a 'representative' panel; it is about constantly reaching out across communities, tapping into the intelligence of individuals and organisations in diverse ways.

The need for more opportunities to share best practice permeates several of the contributions. While many also suggest the importance of more specific guidance, a central message from this book is that there is no 'one best way' of involving patients and the public. Furthermore, there is much that can be done within existing resource constraints.

New information technologies offer previously unthinkable opportunities to tap the local population's views in accessible outlets. Some PCG/Ts are exploring the potential of new polling methodologies using terminals placed in libraries, supermarkets and health service premises. Digital TV opens up future possibilities of rapid access to health advice and information at home 24 hours a day. These new services will complement the NHS Direct telephone helpline, NHS on-line and other sources of rapid access to primary care including walk-in centres (Figure C.1).

An extended range of channels offers the possibility of targeted support to specific groups such as patients with chronic ailments and their carers. Possible health applications for digital TV are listed in Table C.1 (Dick, 2000). Creative use of information technology, particularly the Internet, both to communicate with patients and to manage patient care, will be central to future clinical practice. Fundamental re-design rather than ever-faster spinning of the 'hamster wheel' of health care may be the only way of sustaining the NHS (Morrison and Smith, 2000).

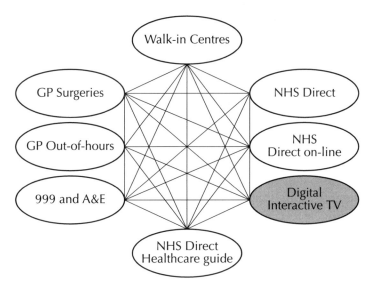

**Figure C.1** Access network for health information and advice and fast primary care (Dick, 2000)

## 4. The need for further research

A particular kind of relationship between health professionals and patients is required if shared decision-making is to take place. Traditional paternalistic relationships are ill-equipped for the task. While in recent years there has been a movement away from paternalistic relationships towards partnerships, they are by no means universal. It is difficult to know what proportion of contacts are 'patient-centred'. Several chapters presented evidence that poor communication is a continuing source of user dissatisfaction. More studies are needed to explore how approaches to shared decision-making affect patient satisfaction or health outcomes.

**Table C.1** Possible health applications for digital TV          (Dick, 2000)

*Support for individuals*

- Individual health information and advice, for example, links to NHS Direct call centres and NHS On-line; to the national electronic library for health and to health authorities.
- Individual diagnosis, treatment and care, for example, telemonitoring, teleconsulting, televisiting (virtual house calls, hospital at home, etc.).
- Administrative services, for example, appointment booking, repeat prescription requests, test results.
- Affinity group support, for example, to patients with chronic conditions and their carers.

*Support to communities*

- Community development, for example, virtual healthy living centres, support to local health action zones, etc.
- NHS news and views, for example, ministerial, chief medical officer and chief nursing officer broadcasts.
- Public consultation, for example, on NHS developments.

*Support to the NHS*

- Professional training and development, for example, on best practice. Staff recruitment such as job advertisements. Research and monitoring, for example, patient surveys.

Florin and Coulter have summarised work already carried out on ways of sharing information with patients. There is, however, scope for further research to explore the range of different strategies that can be used in the consultation and, in particular, to define when shared decision-making is appropriate. We also need to know more about current professional and user relationships. What expectations do professionals and patients have of each other? What concerns them most and leads them to criticise each other for inappropriate behaviour? What are professional and consumer groups doing now to bring about improvements? Such research would be an important acknowledgement of the barriers to user involvement. It is likely to have significant implications for both doctors and patients in terms of training and the acceptance of new responsibilities.

## 5. Commitment, not techniques

While it is important to be clear about aims, audiences, timing and methods, these contributors do not get hung-up on techniques. That there are differing views on how to involve the public is no excuse for inaction. The evidence base for many health service activities is similarly weak. Inaction is more often due to cultural resistance and lack of confidence than to a shortage of resources or guidance on methods. The methods are not an end in themselves but a statement of organisational values. It is usually better to do something rather than nothing as long as learning is shared. Moreover, few of the contributors are starry-eyed about user involvement for it involves risk taking. Tensions, conflict – and sometimes failure – have to be openly acknowledged. In short, we need 'good enough' public involvement.

## Moving forward

Policy-makers are understandably as ambivalent about user involvement as those working at other levels of the service, as the consultation over *The NHS Plan* indicated. While preaching the rhetoric of user involvement and local autonomy, this government has been no less centralising in many respects than its predecessors. The imposition of a universal model for primary care commissioning and a host of new bodies designed to standardise treatment in the NHS are testimony to this. Government needs to lead debate about the ethical trade-offs involved in resource allocation – to promote frameworks for decision-making – if public expectations are to be re-aligned and commitment to the founding principles of the NHS is to be reaffirmed (Berwick, 1997).

There is as yet little evidence that the 'New NHS' is engaging users more effectively, either in the identification of local service priorities or the implementation of clinical governance. PCG/Ts are struggling to engage their publics in their work. The role of the lay member is an ambiguous one. How effective will they be at promoting the requisite cultural change?

The new Patient Advocacy and Liaison Service and associated advisory forums provide a characteristically structural solution to the shortcomings of the Community Health Councils they replace.

As Anderson argues, the Government risks creating apparatus that serves principally to legitimate the vested interests of clinicians and managers. This risk can be reduced if an effective mix of patient and public involvement methods is in place locally. Such involvement should be pursued in partnership with local authorities and voluntary organisations, for any engagement with users about their health exposes the irrelevance to individuals of institutional boundaries. Most crucially, user involvement must be linked to organisational change. Visible mechanisms are less important than their impact at every level of the service – on strategic decision-making, operational planning and professional practice.

Since the Alma-Ata Declaration, international observers have offered a vision of primary health care as transcending a curative model of health services (MacDonald, 1993). Instead, primary health care, it is claimed, offers the potential for a people-orientated approach that acknowledges the holistic nature of health (Coombs, 1997). British primary medical care remains far from the WHO model in certain respects. Current challenges in the form of a changing policy and organisational environment present opportunities for dialogue about the nature of primary care in the UK (NHS Executive, 1998). A central message from the case studies is that user involvement not only initiates dialogue but is indeed a means to achieve change.

The challenges raised in this book are not amenable to solution in the usual sense. Instead, they help understand the task ahead. This text was never intended to be a 'DIY manual', but if it provides reassurance about what counts as progress, realism about what can be expected, and encouragement to invest energy in some of the approaches described here, a valuable purpose will have been served.

# References

Barnes M, Wistow G. *Researching User Involvement*. Leeds: Nuffield Institute for Health Studies, University of Leeds, 1992.

Beresford P, Croft S, Evans C, Harding T. Quality in personal social services: The developing role of user involvement in the UK. In: Davies C, Finlay L, Bullman A, editors. *Changing practice in health and social care*. London: Sage, 2000.

Berwick D, Hiatt H, Janeway P, Smith R. An ethical code for everyone in health care. *BMJ* 1997; 315: 1633–34.

Bowling A. Health care rationing: the public's debate. *BMJ* 1996; 312: 670–74.

Brambleby P, editor. *Needs Assessment De-Mystified.* Norwich: Norfolk Public Health Nurses Forum, 2000.

Coombes Y. An international perspective on primary health care. In: Sidell M, Jones, L, Katz J, Peberdy A, editors. *Debates and dilemmas in promoting health.* London: Macmillan, 1997.

Department of Health. 'People and Communities'@ohn.gov.uk

Dick P. Screen and heard. *Health Service Journal* 2000; 5 Oct: 37.

NHS Executive. *The NHS Plan. A plan for investment. A plan for reform.* Cm 4818-I. London: The Stationery Office, 2000.

Macdonald, J. *Primary health care. Medicine in its place.* London: Earthscan Publications, 1993.

Morrison J, Smith R. Hamster health care. *BMJ* 2000; 321: 1541–42.

Seymour J. Patient Counselling. *Health Management* 1997; June: 14–17.

Slowie D F. Doctors should help patients to communicate better with them. *BMJ* 1999; 319: 784.

Smith R, Hiatt H, Berwick D. Shared ethical principles for everyone in health care: a working draft from the Tavistock Group. *BMJ* 1999; 318: 248–51.

Stronks K, Strijbis A-M, Wendte J F, Gunning-Schepers L. Who should decide? Qualitative analysis of panel data from public, patients, healthcare professionals, and insurers on priorities in health care. *BMJ* 1997; 315: 92–96.

Wright A. Exploring the development of user forums in an NHS trust. In: Barnes M, Warren L, editors. *Paths to empowerment.* Bristol: The Policy Press, 1999.

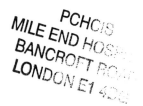